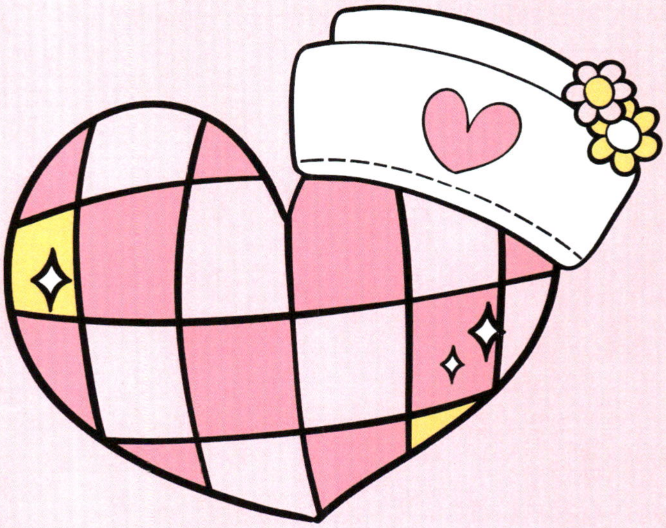

This notebook belongs to:

___

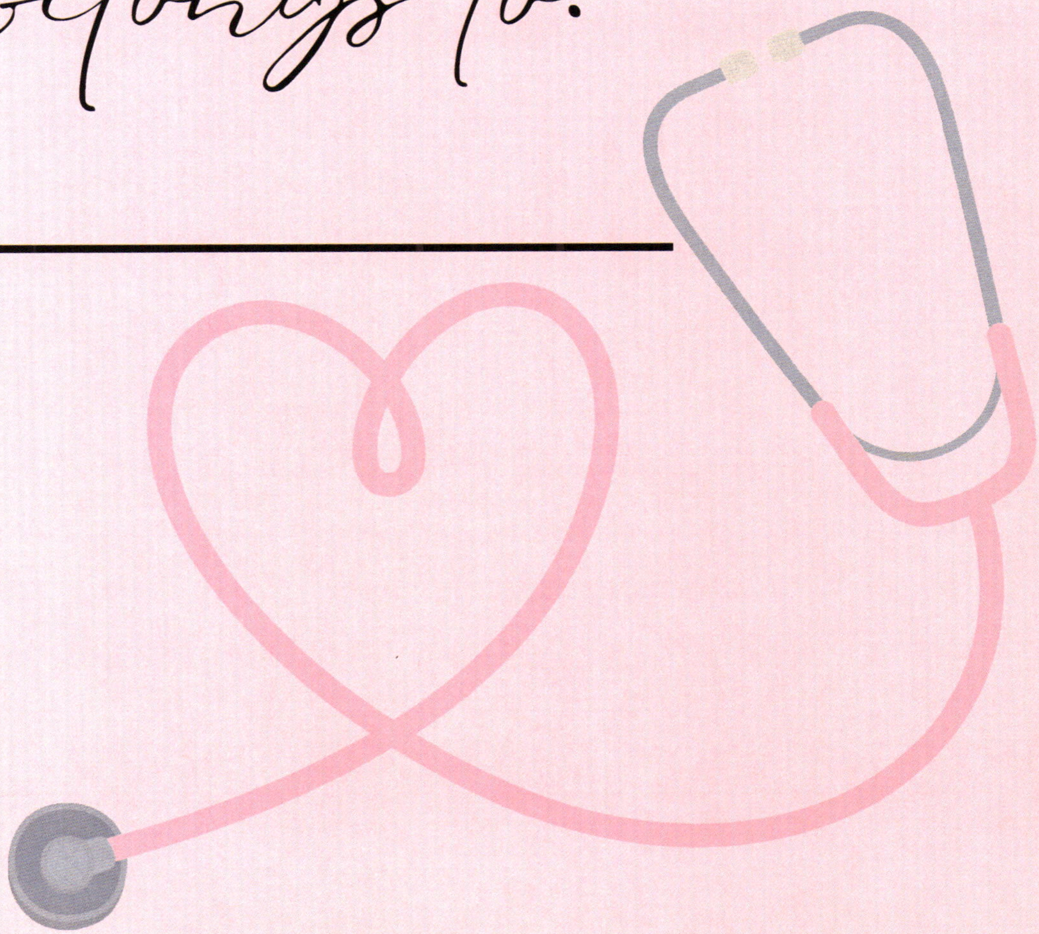

Prayer for Nurses

May your loving hands touch the hearts of your patients. You are the hands & feet of Christ. You will share laughter and tears with your patients. Don't be afraid to share the love of God. Each encounter may be your last.

Maria Flores

Touch the Heart

NURSE

NOTEBOOK

BY: MARIA A FLORES

Touch the Heart, Reach the Soul LLC
Polk City, FL, USA

Touch the Heart Nurse Notebook

Faith Based Journals, Coloring Books, Planners, Notebooks, Home Decor, Apparel & Gift Items
http://touchtheheartreachthesoul.store

Manuscript, design, illustrations, and book cover by Maria A Flores

http://touchtheheartreachthesoul.store
customerservice@touchtheheartreachthesoul.com

Nurse

Nurse

Nurse

NURSE

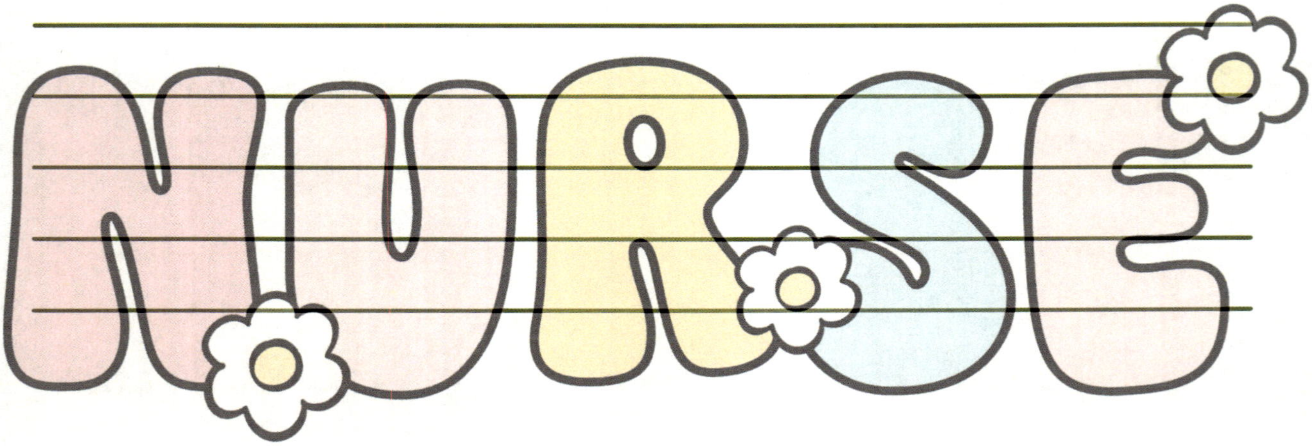
NURSE

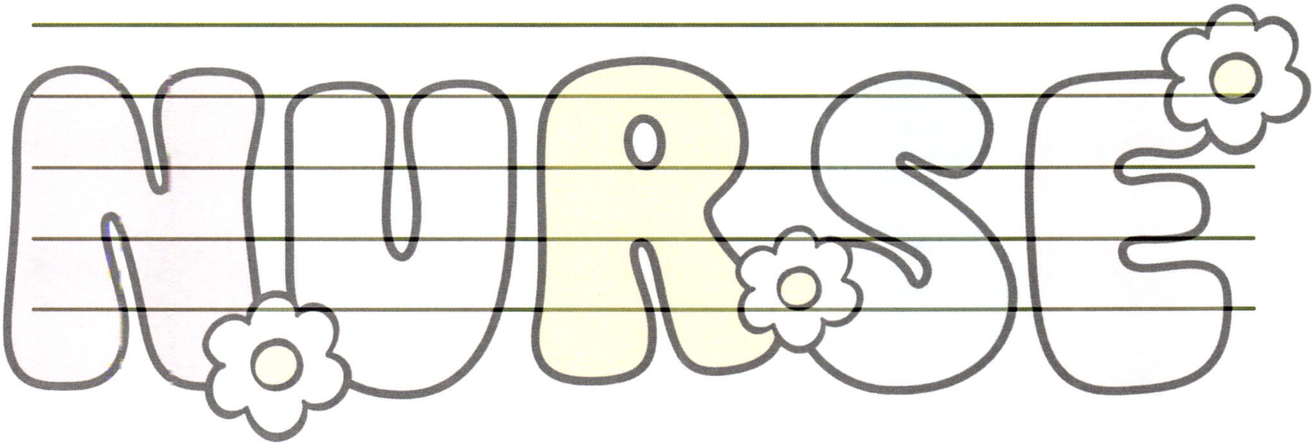
NURSE

NURSE

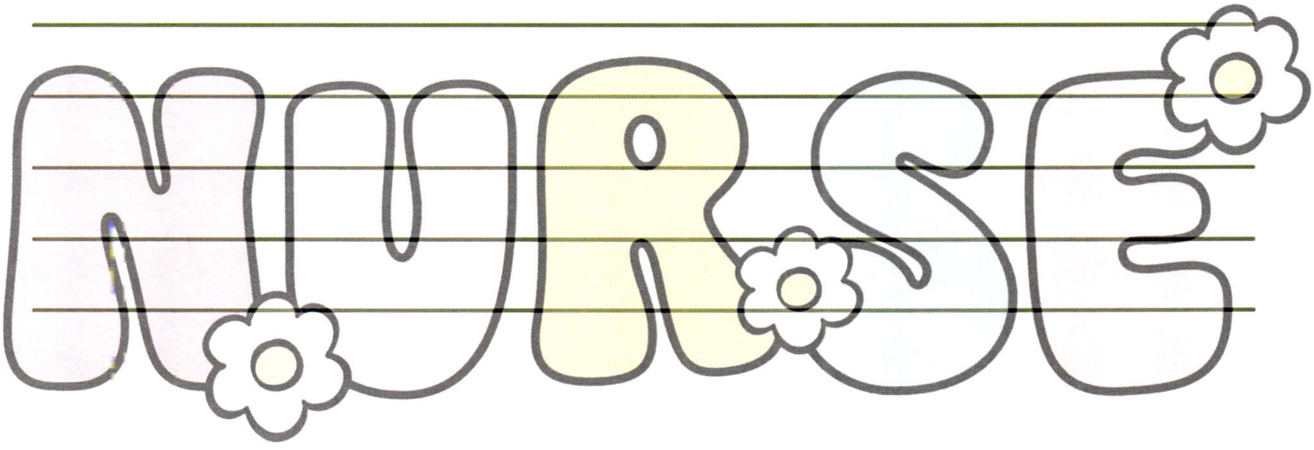
NURSE

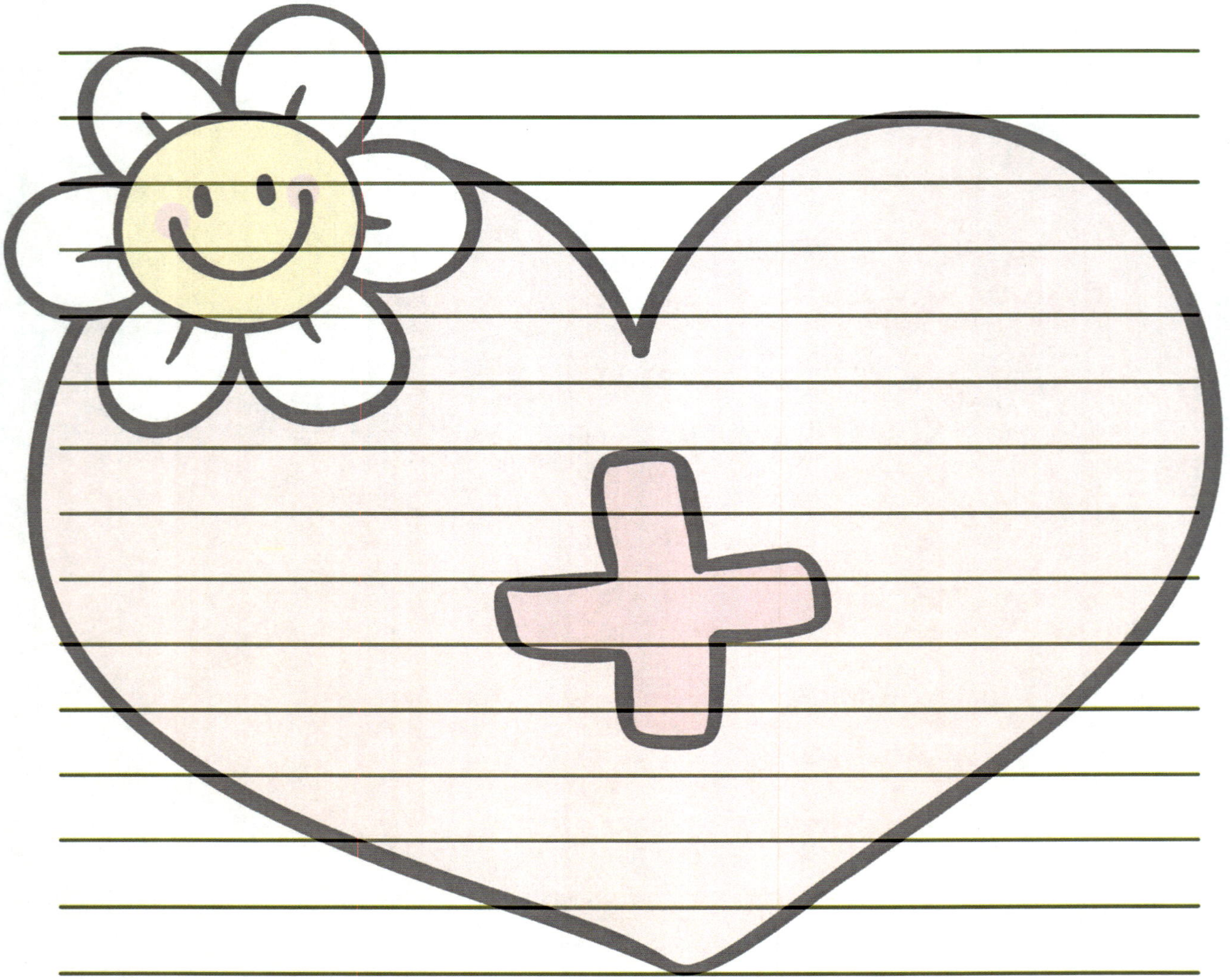

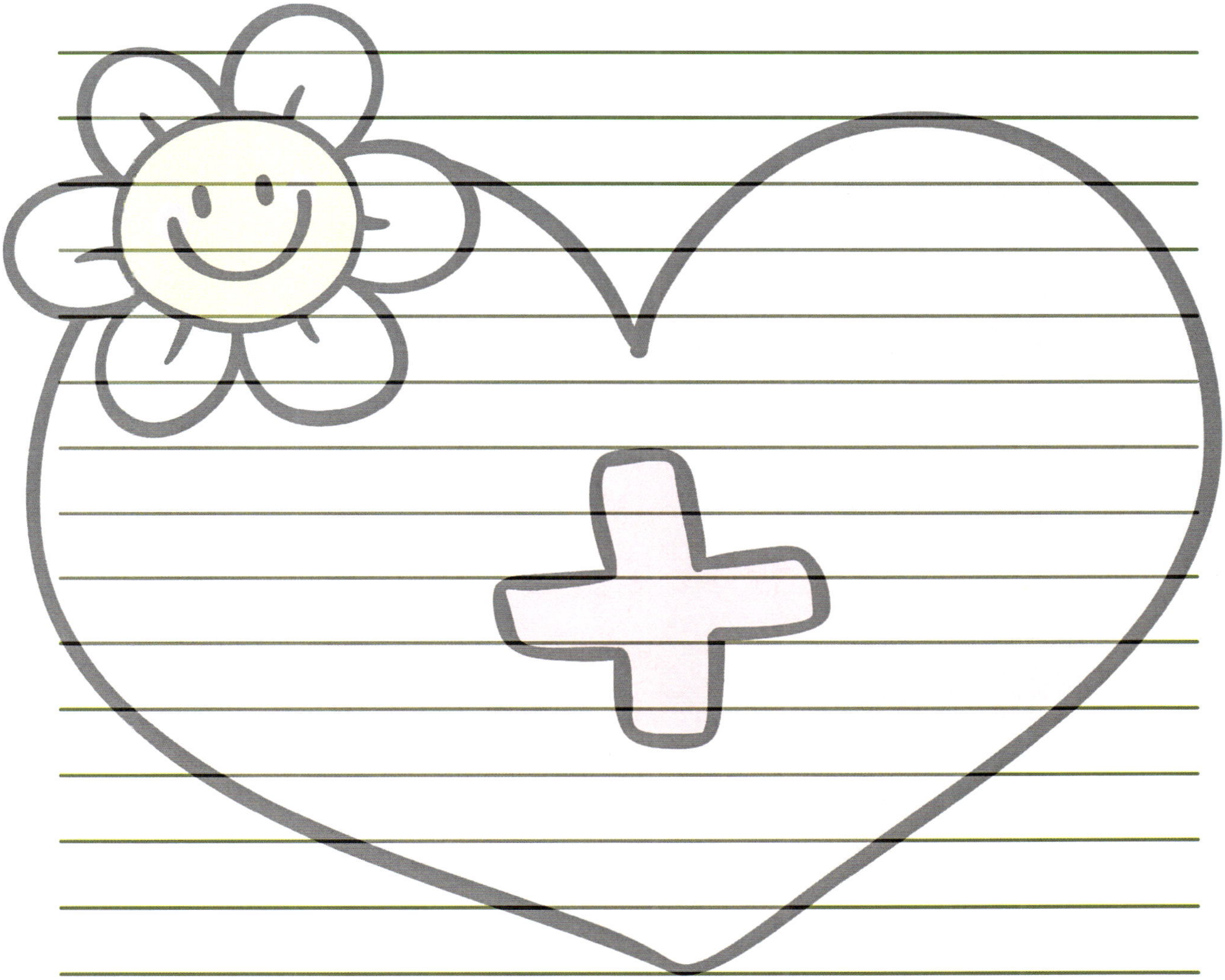

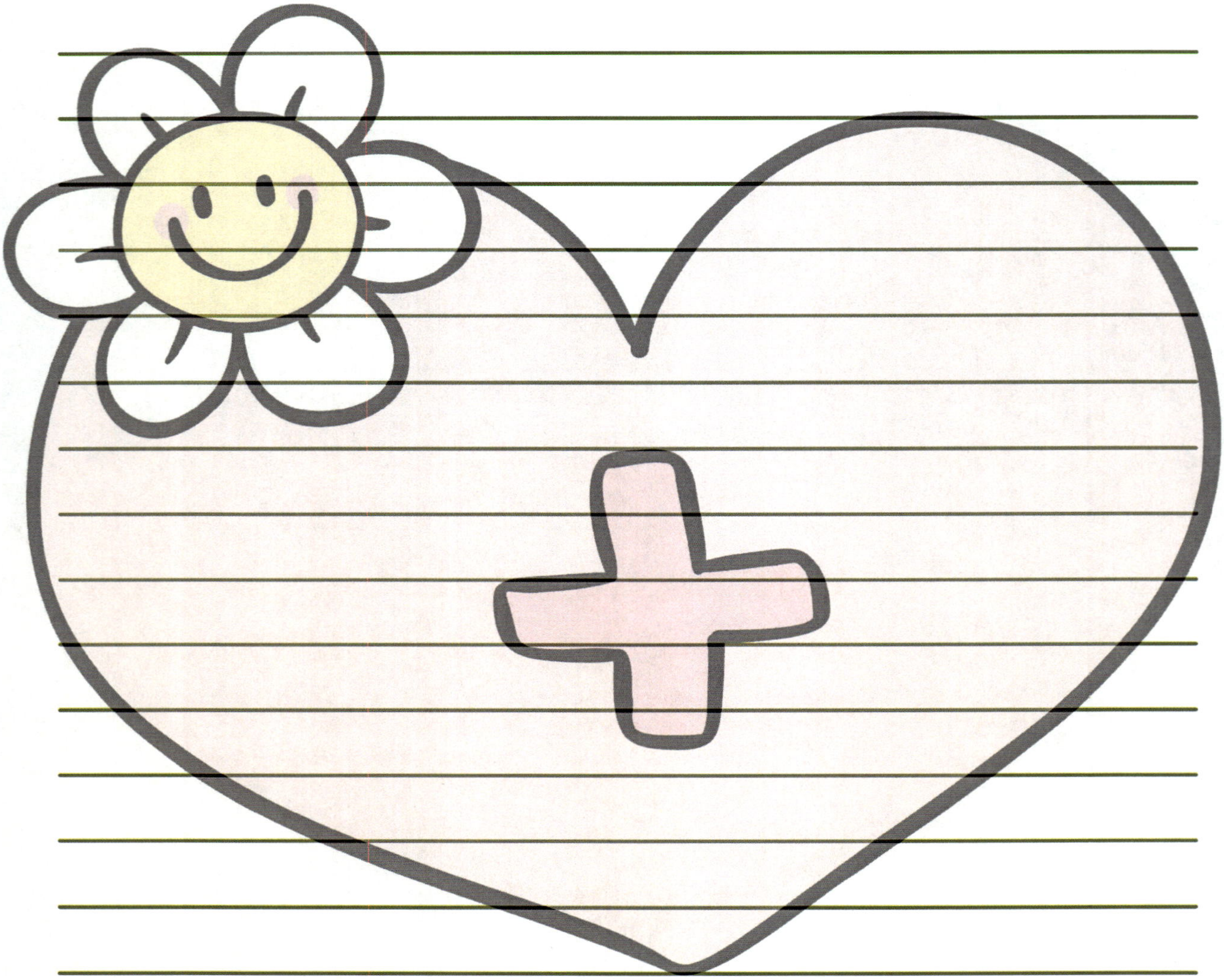

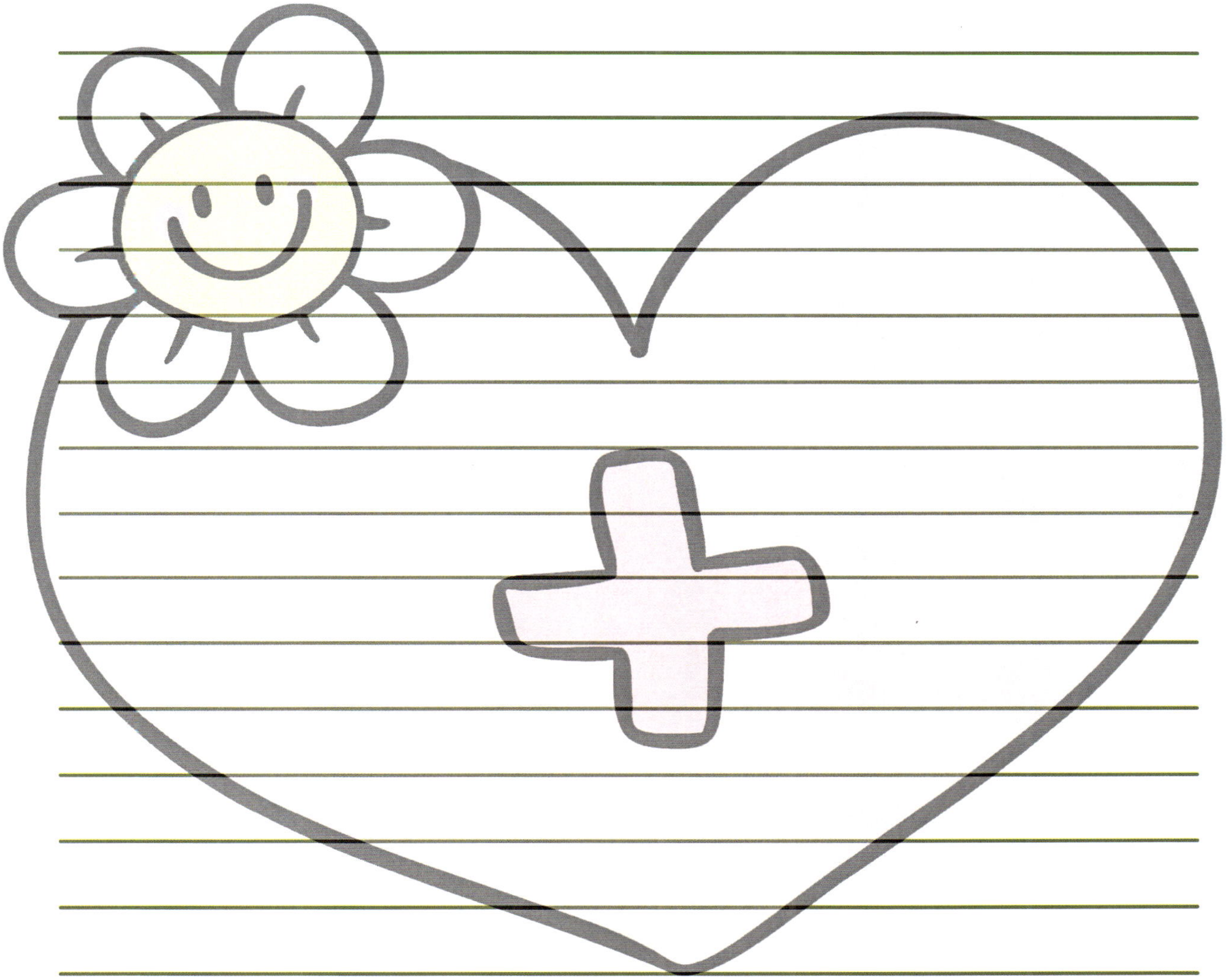

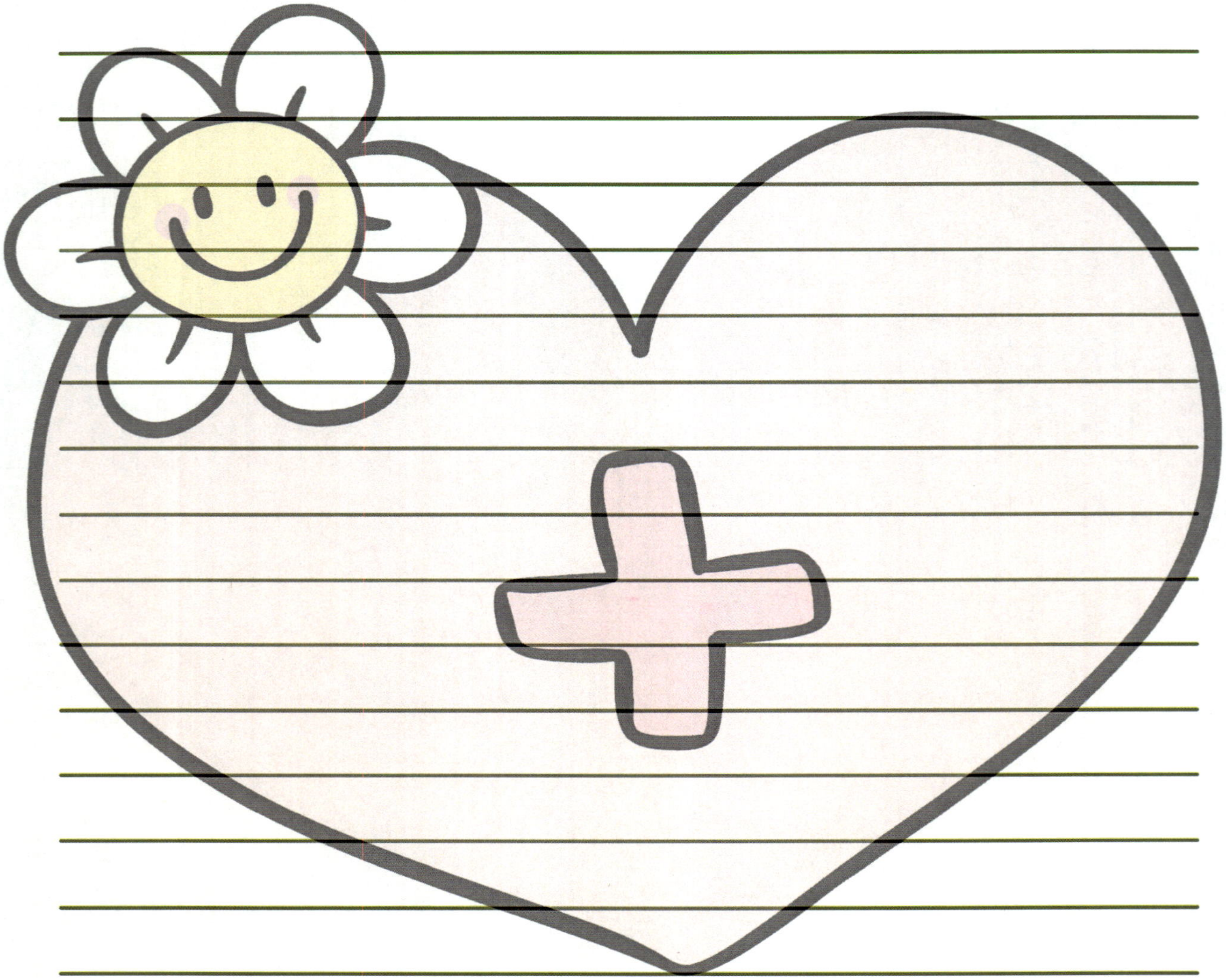

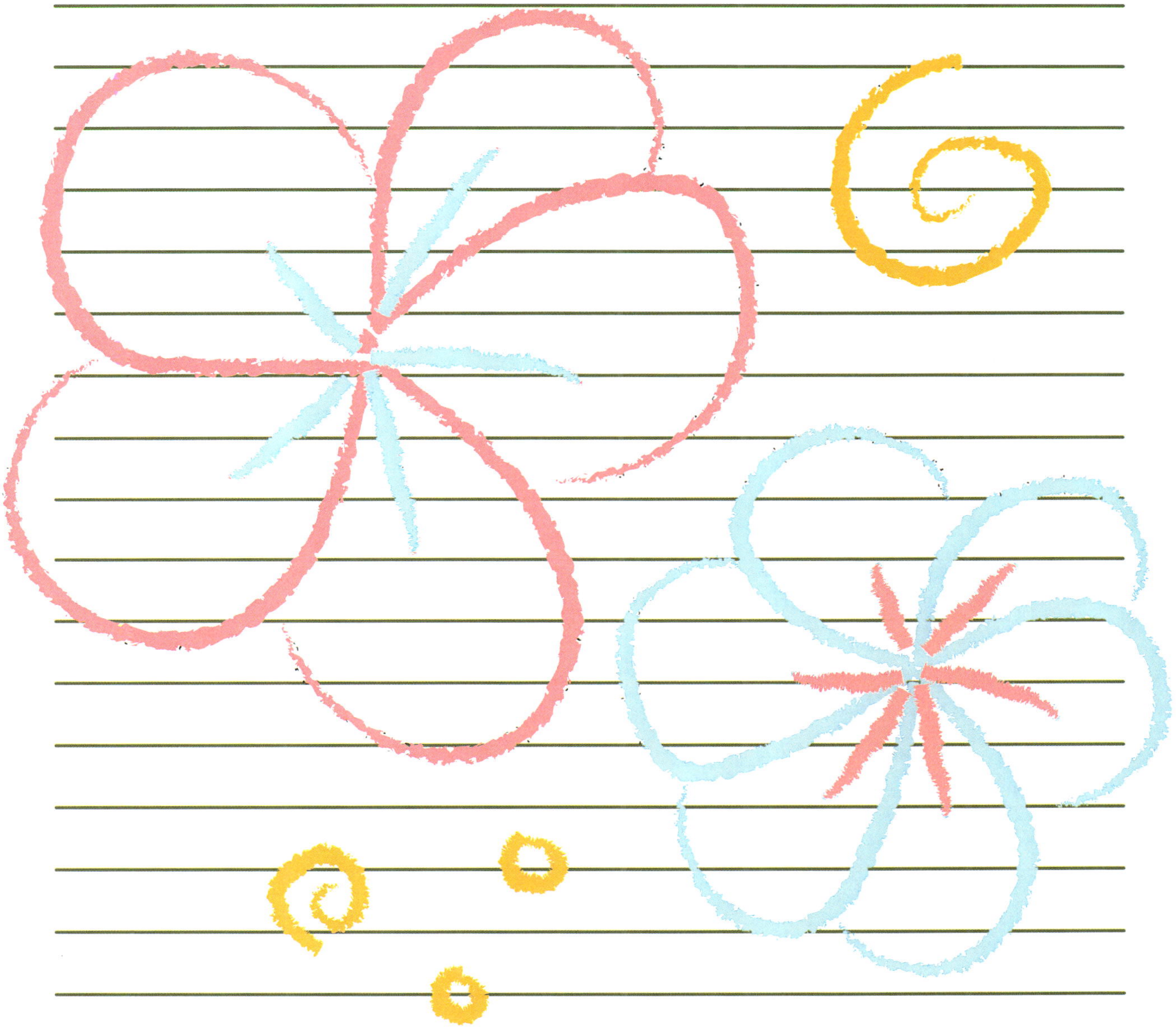

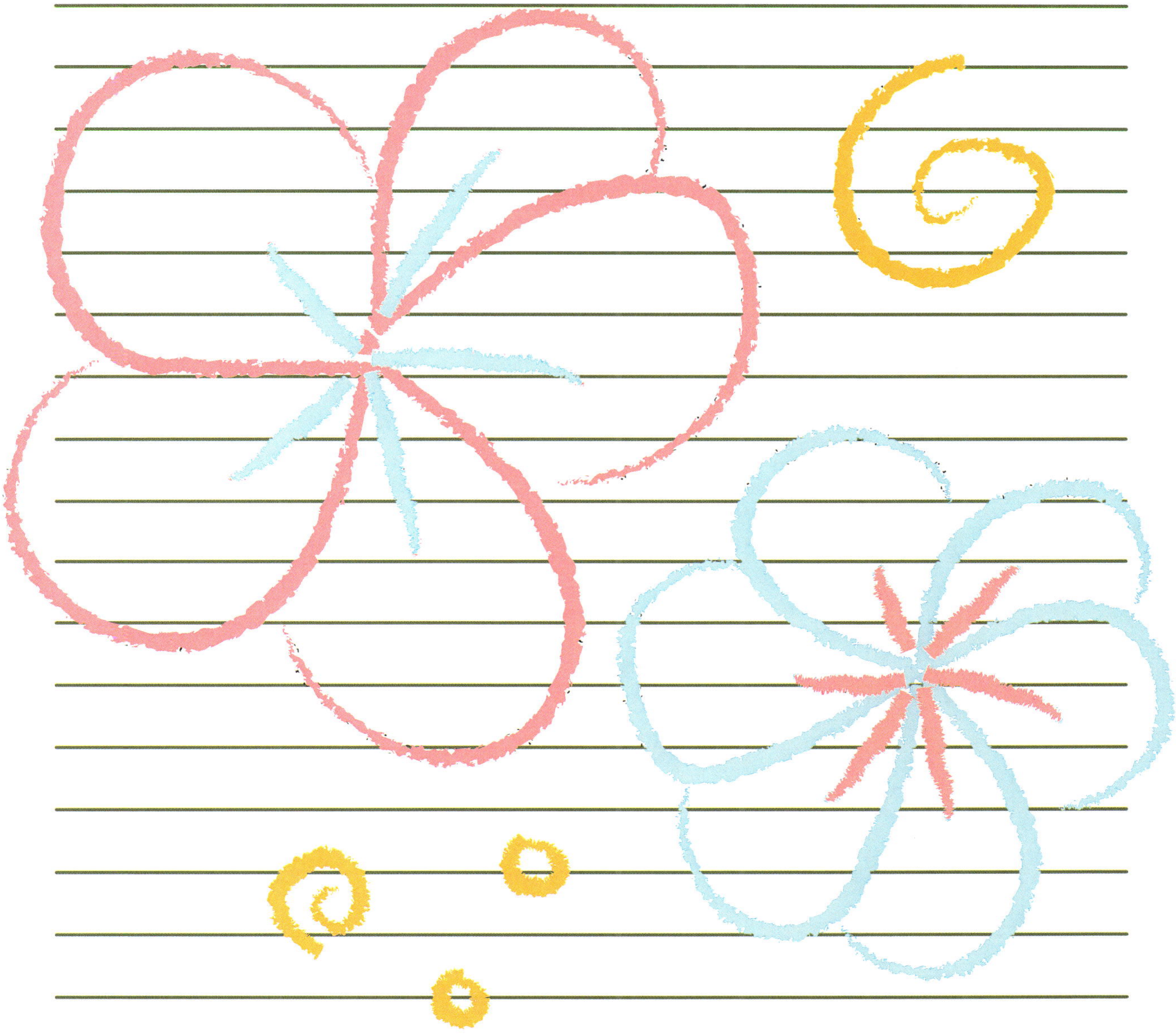

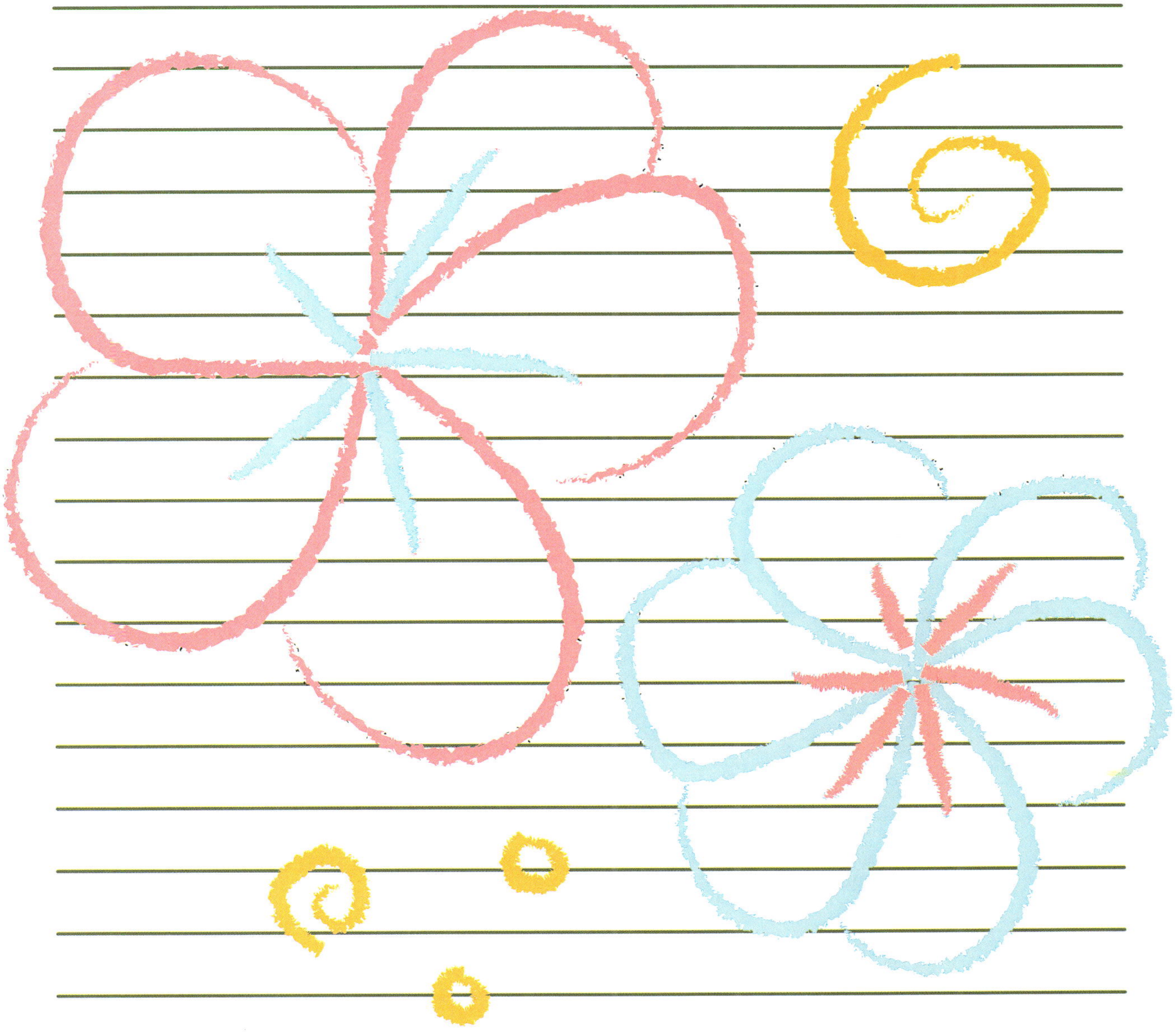

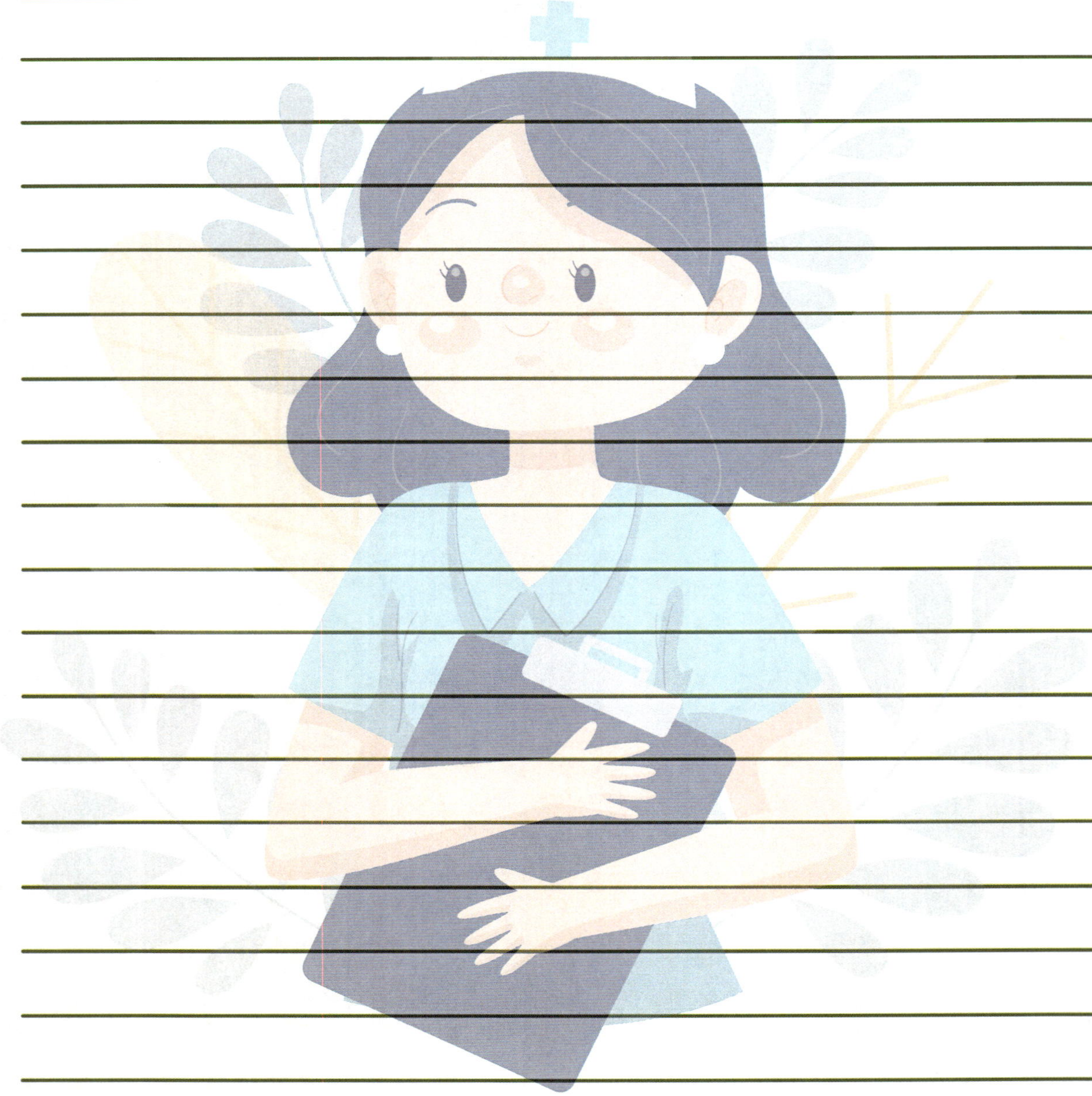

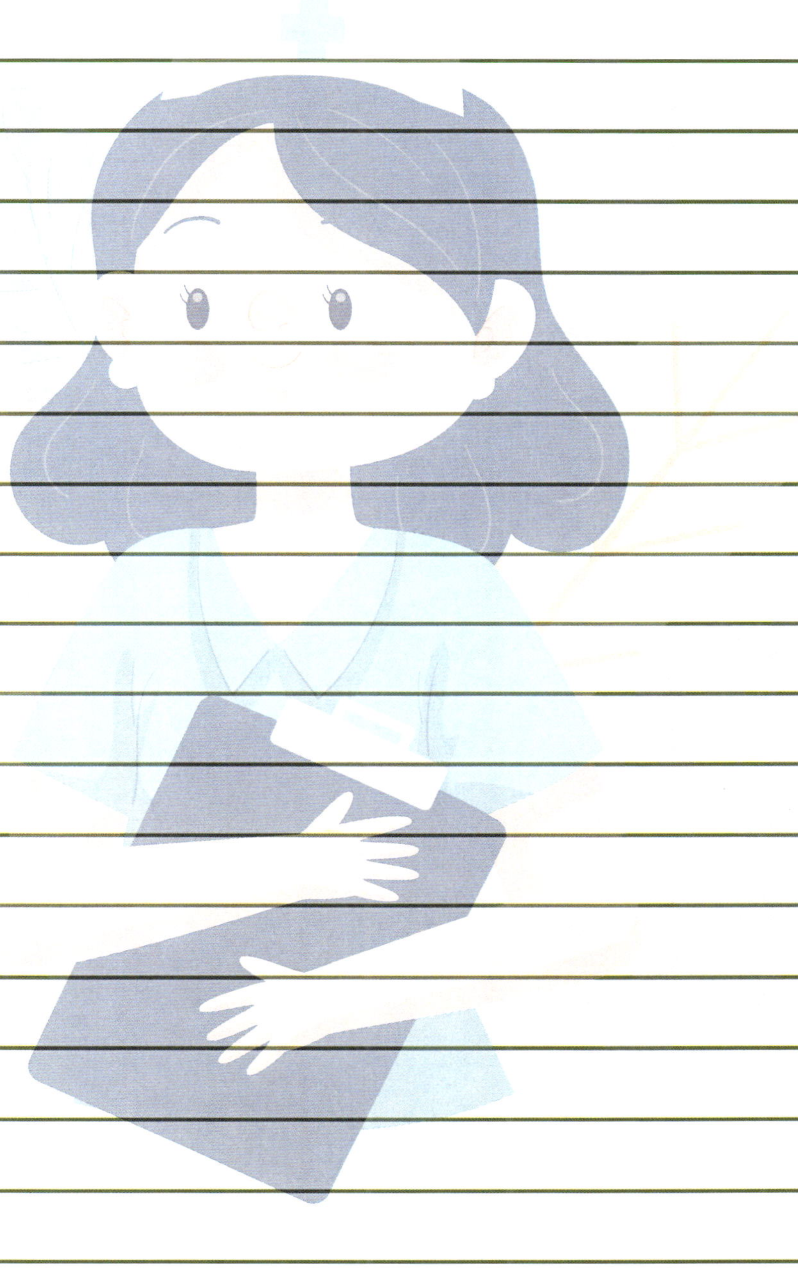

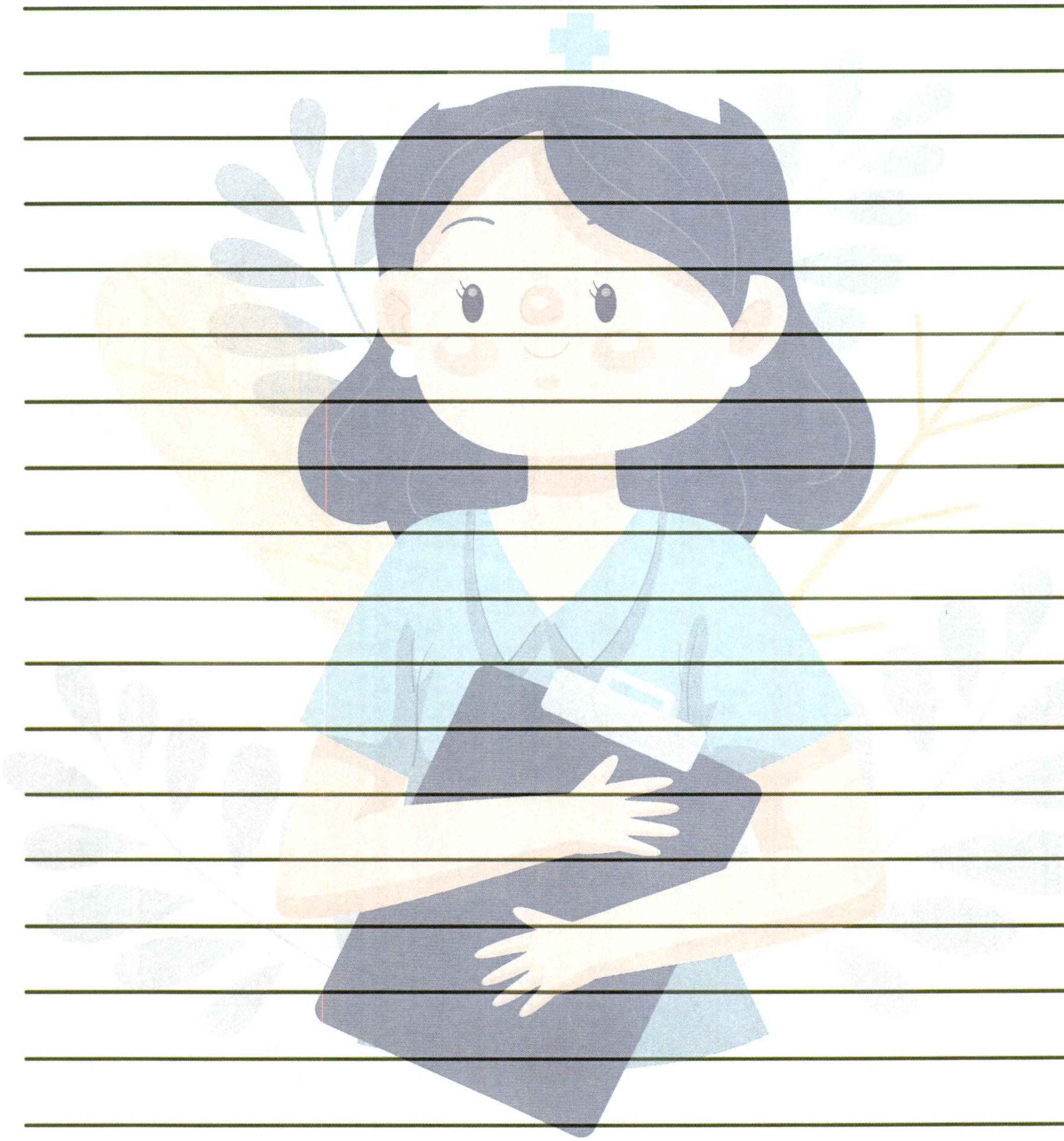

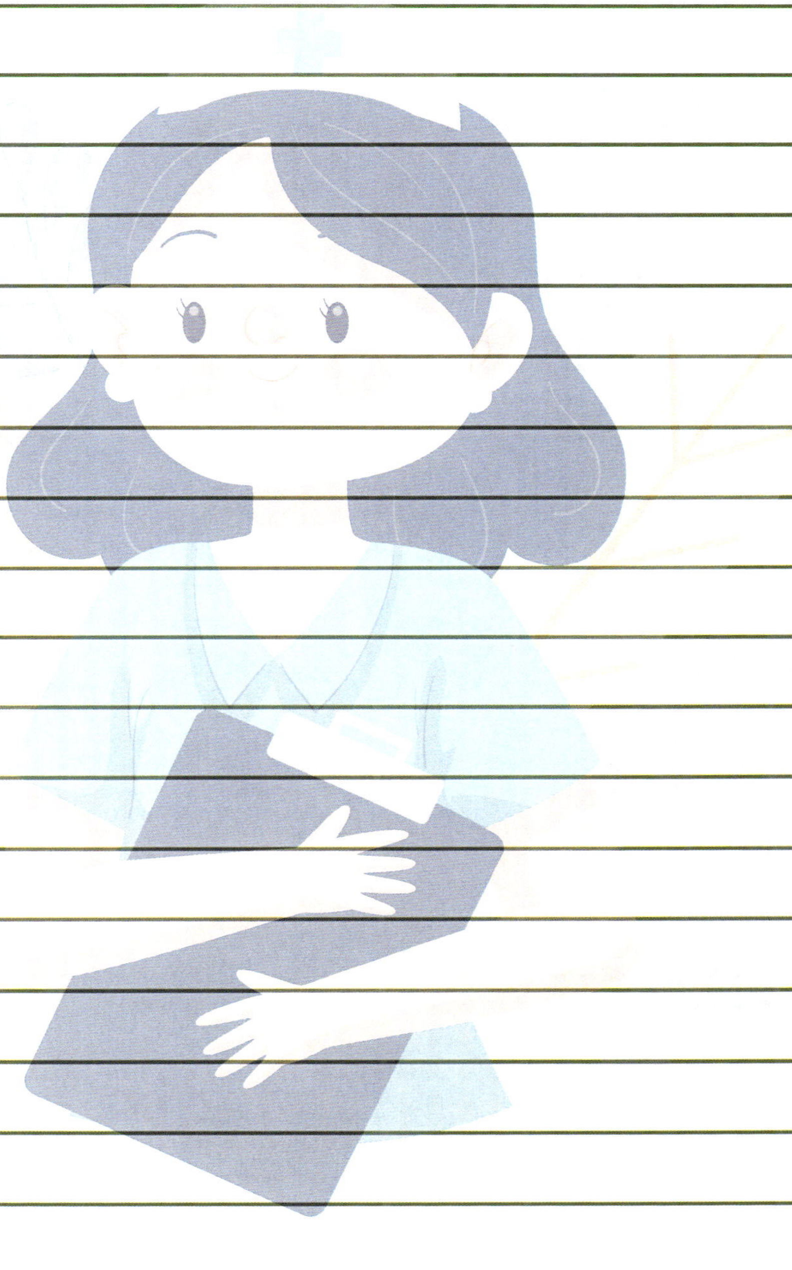

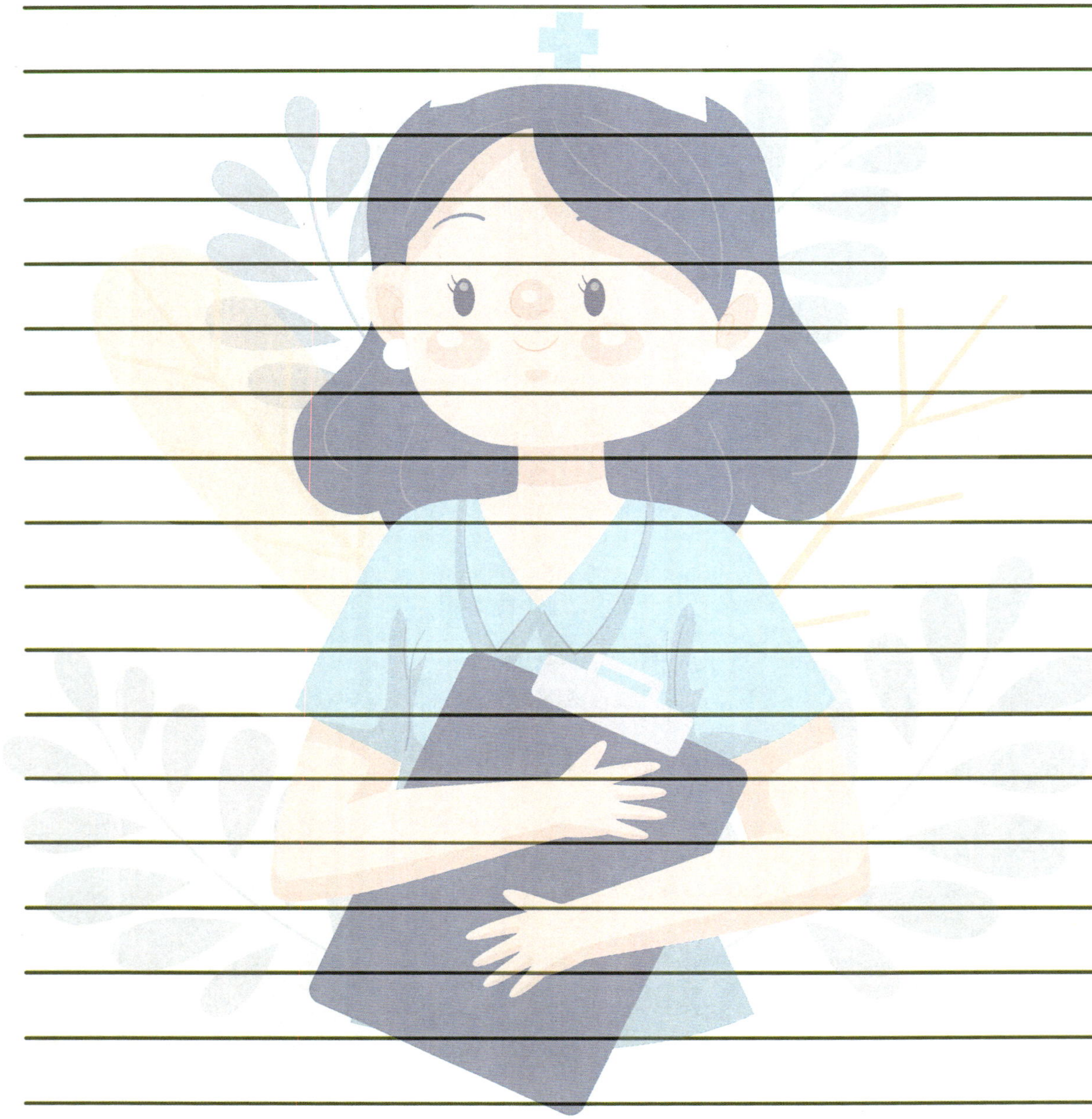

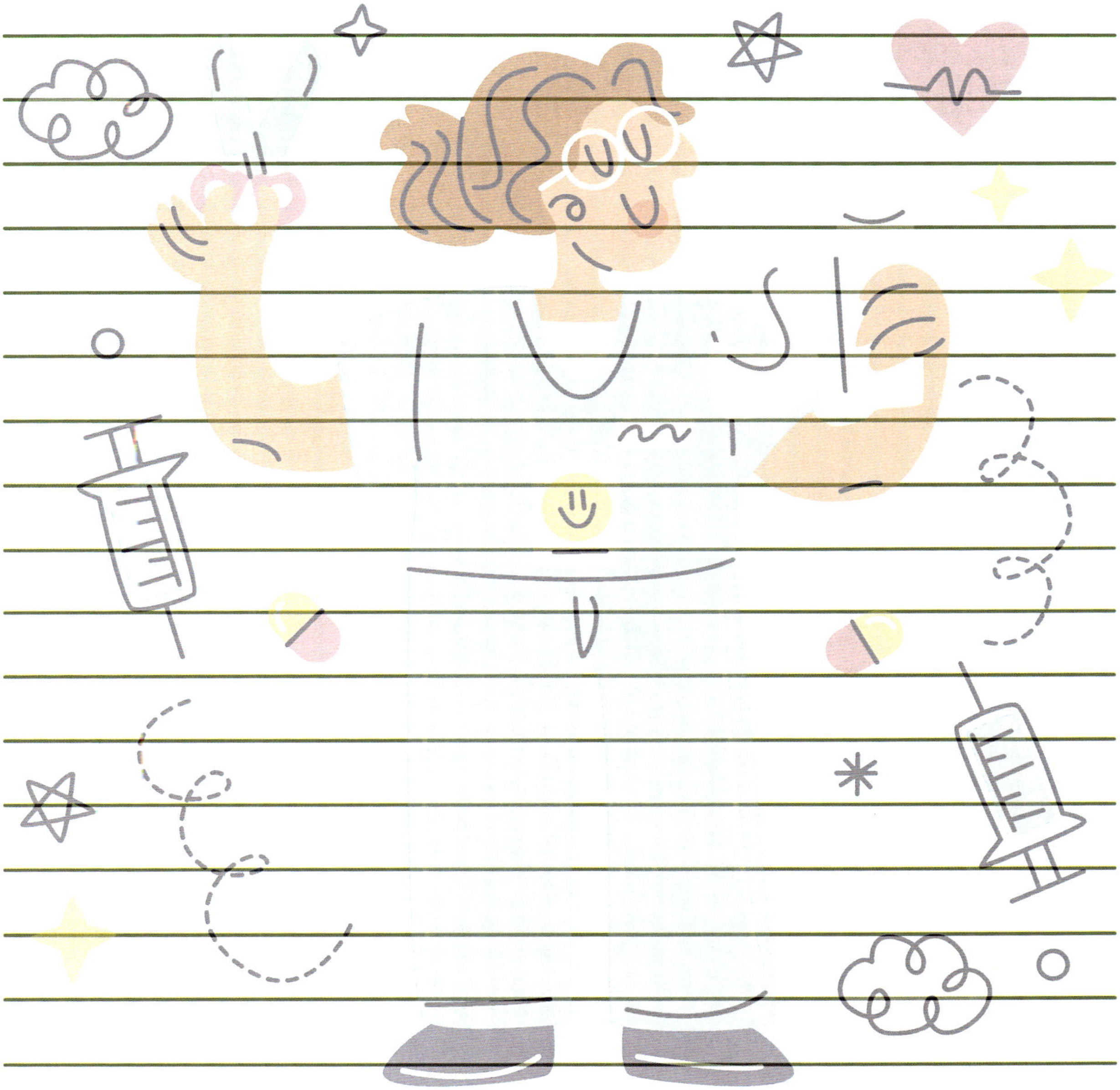

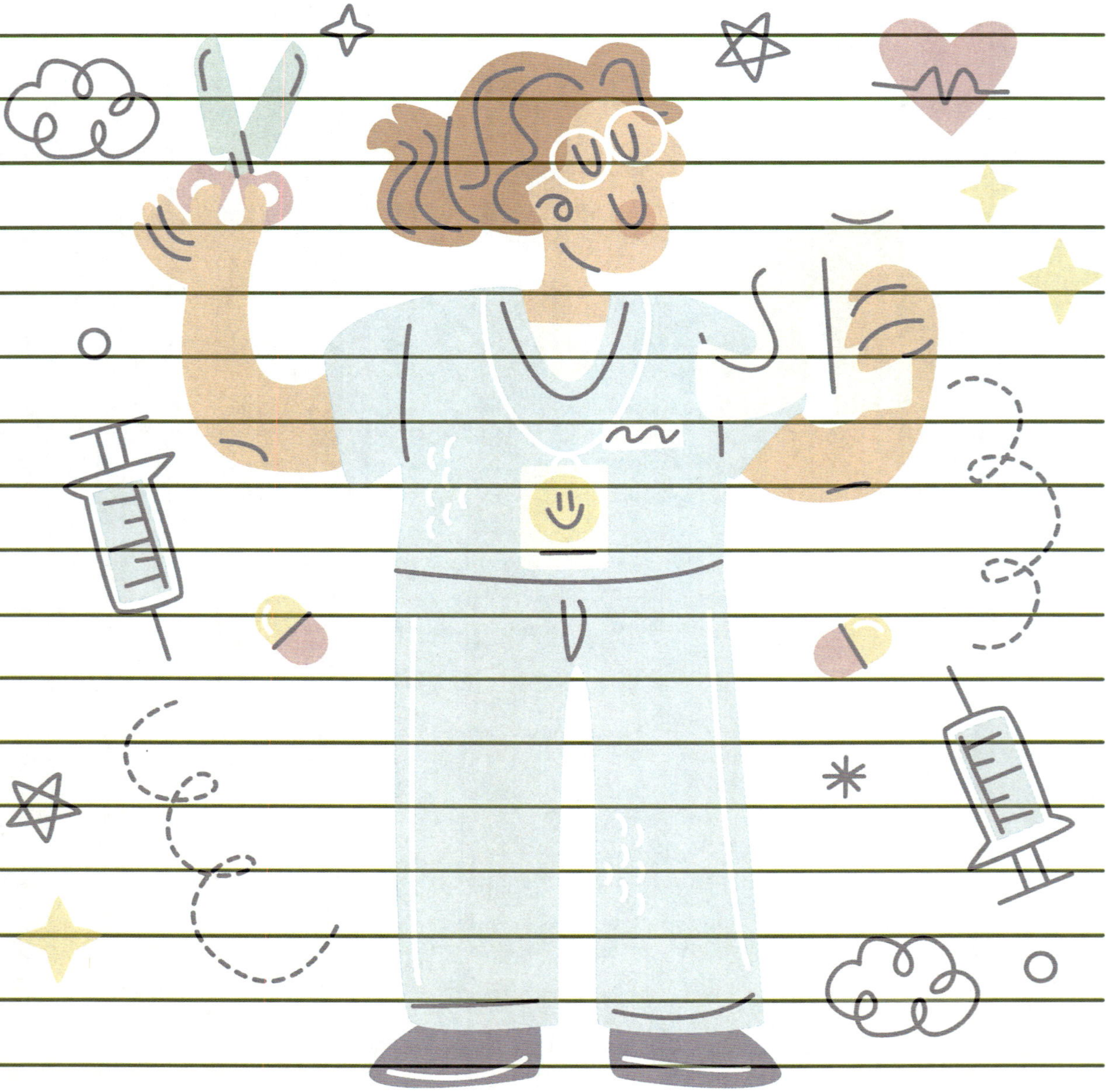

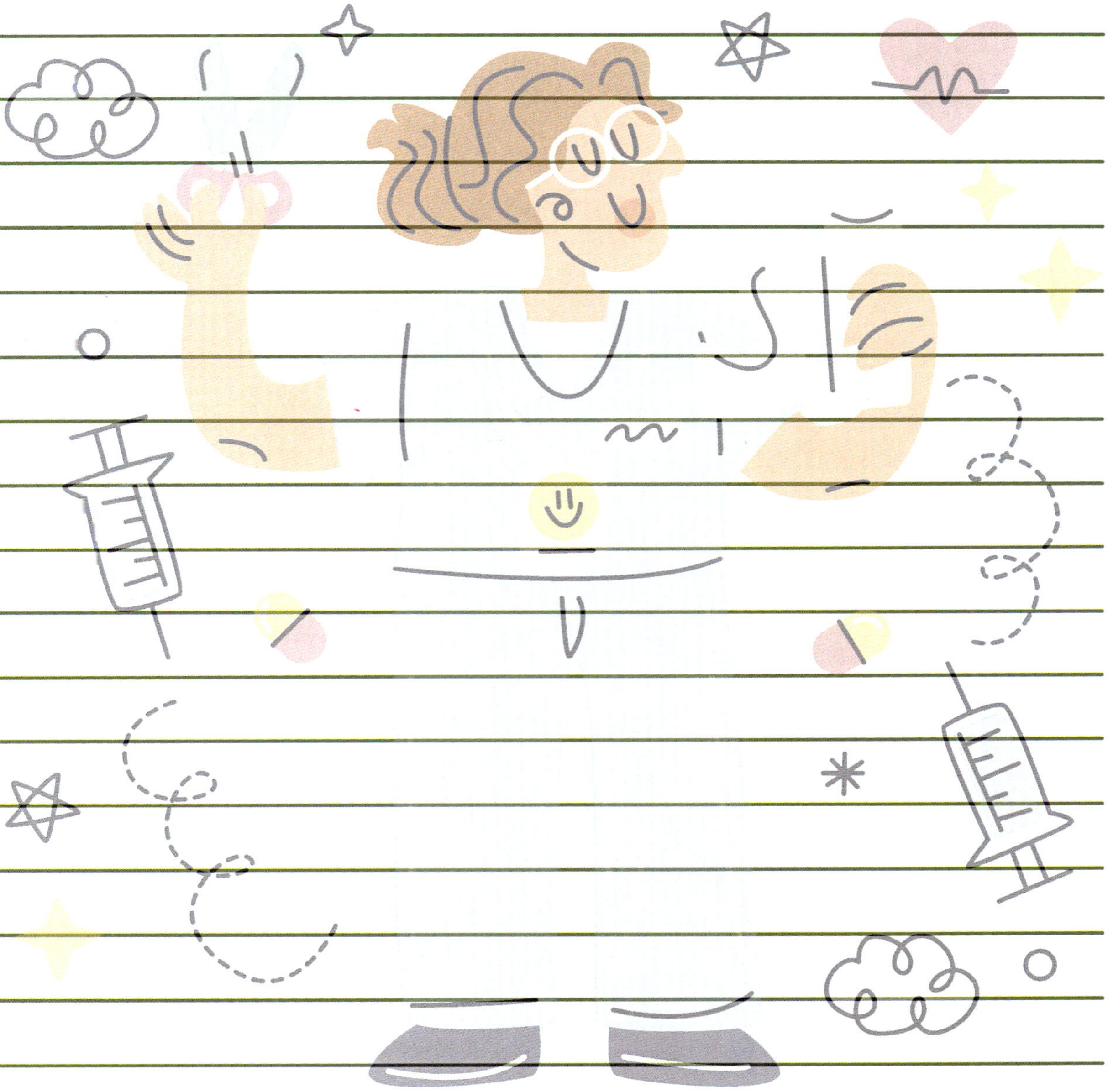

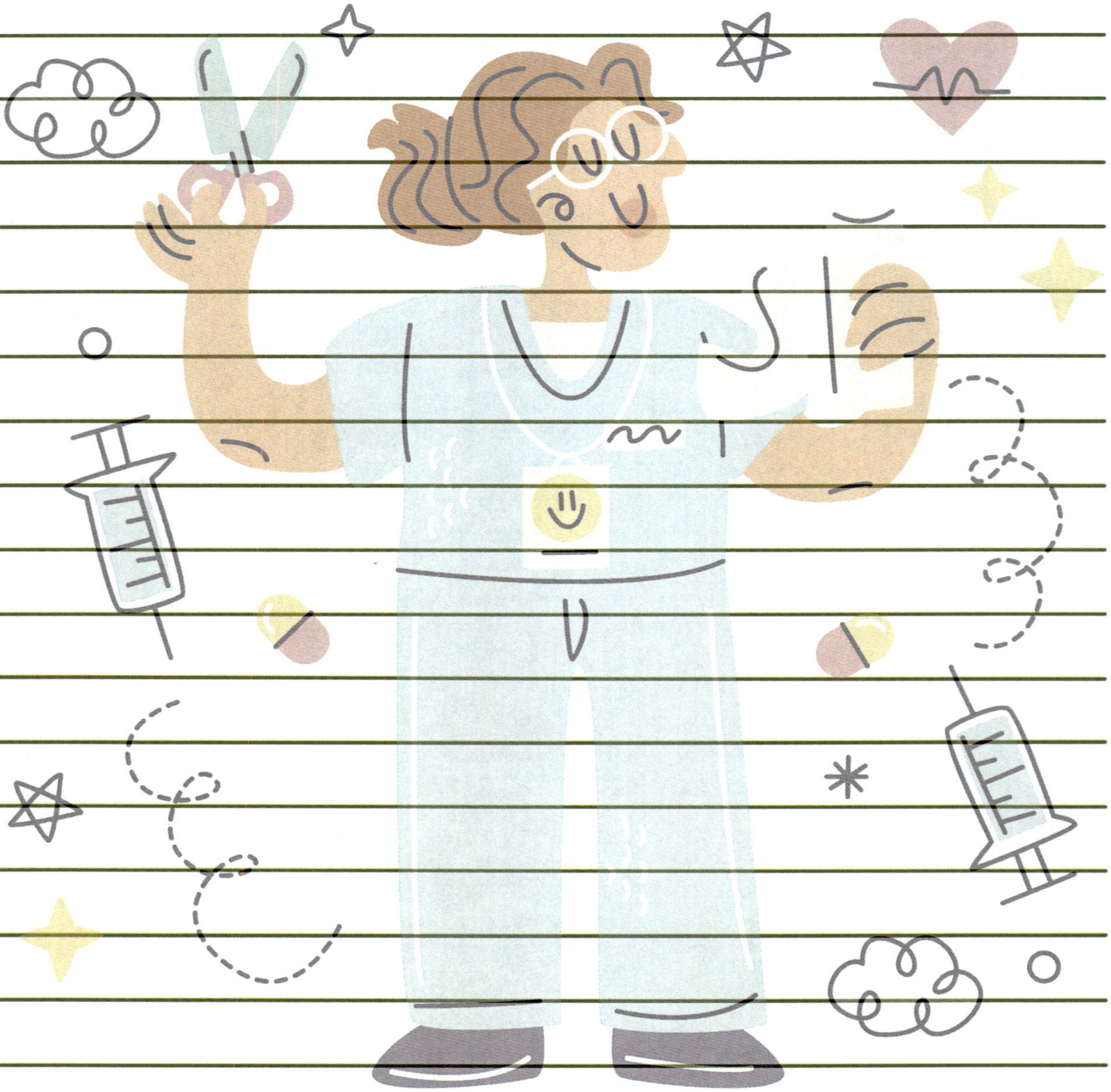

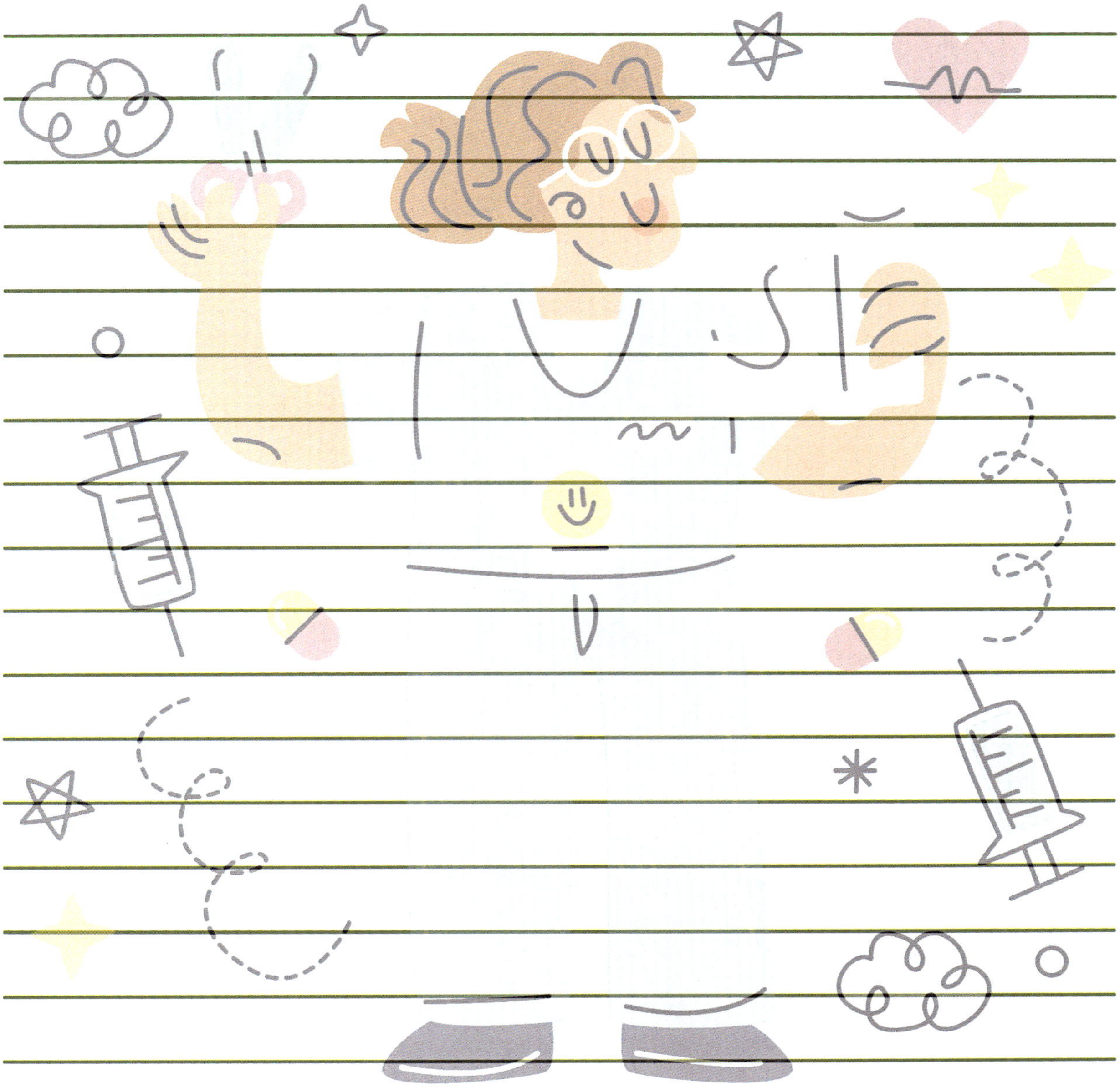

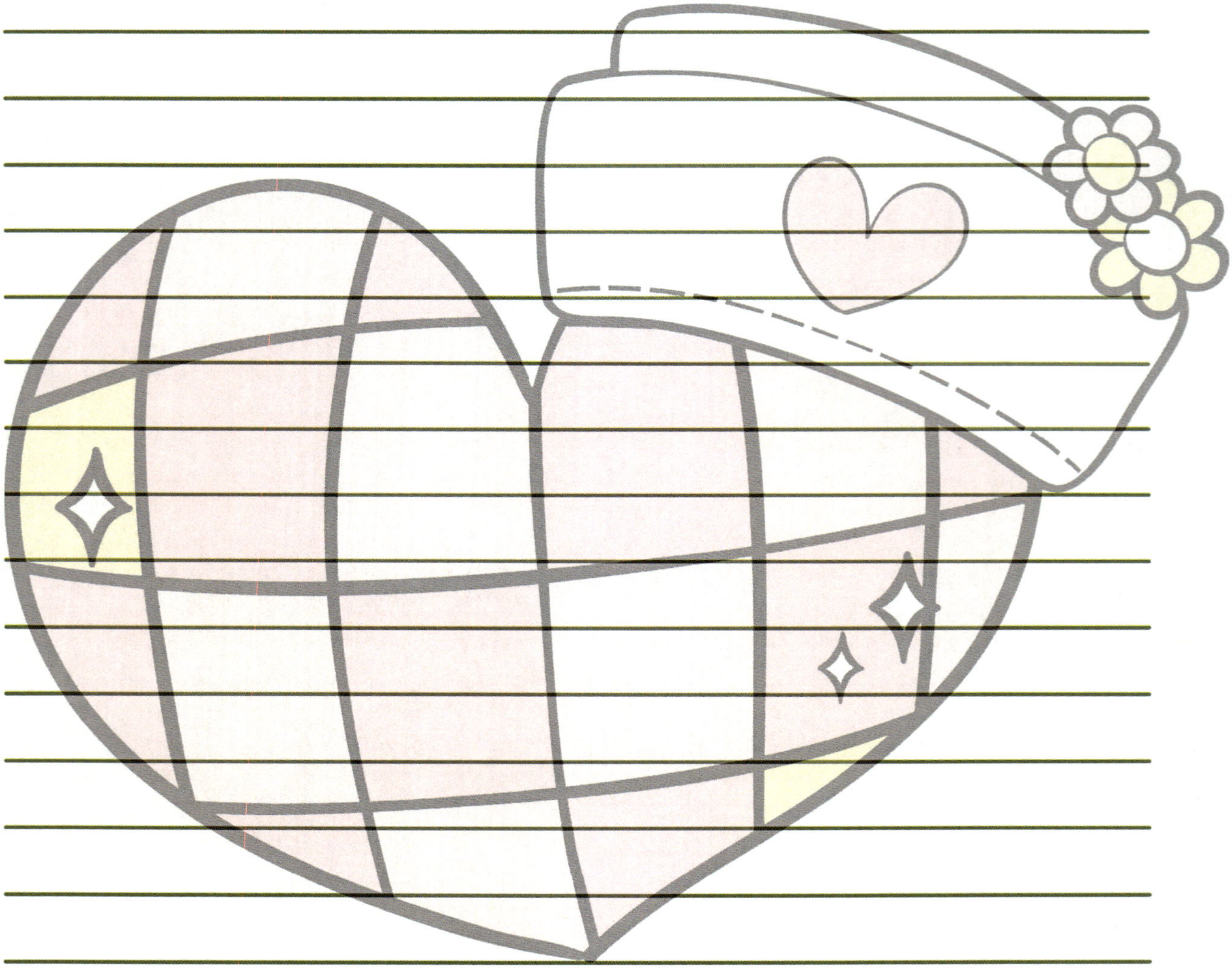

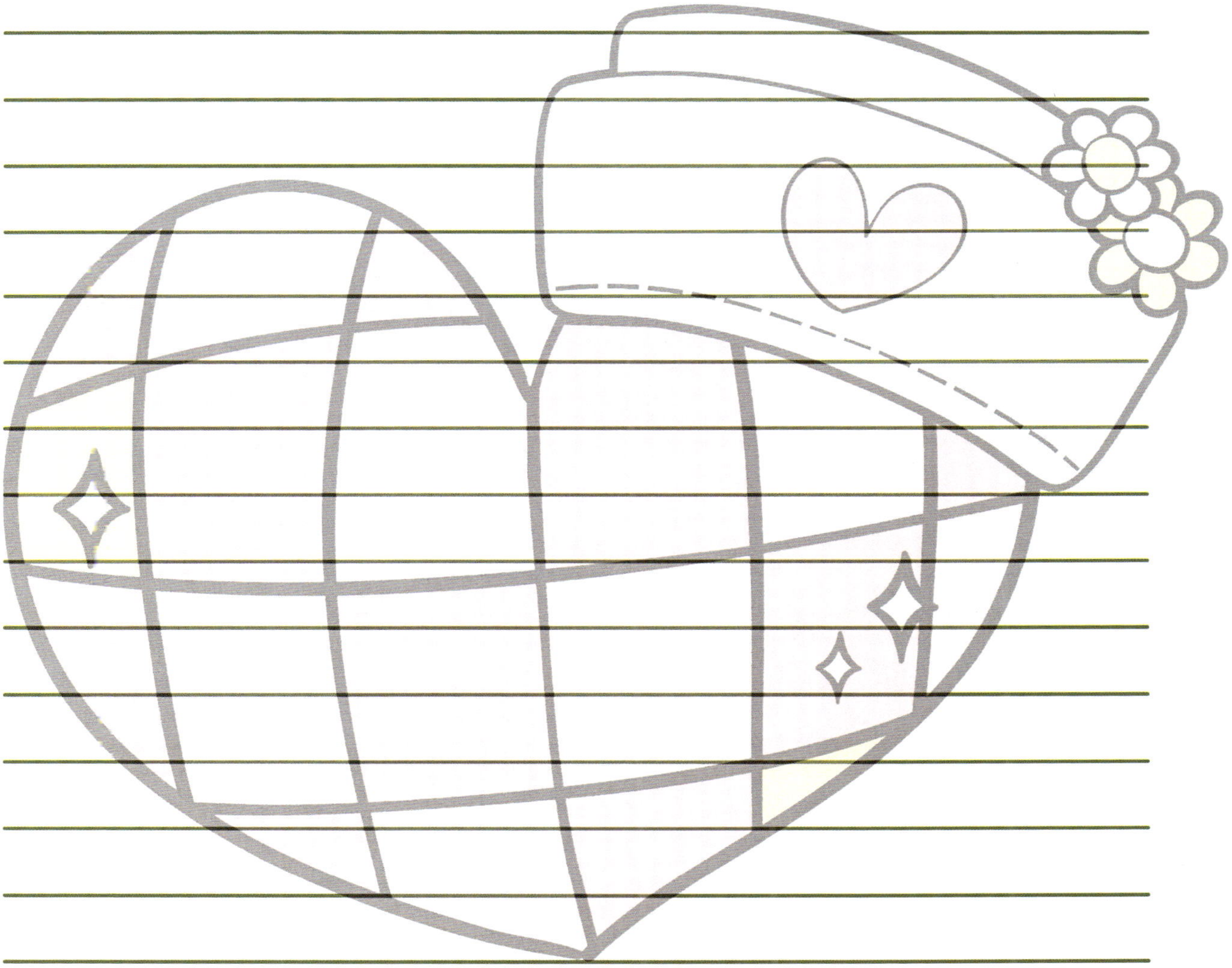

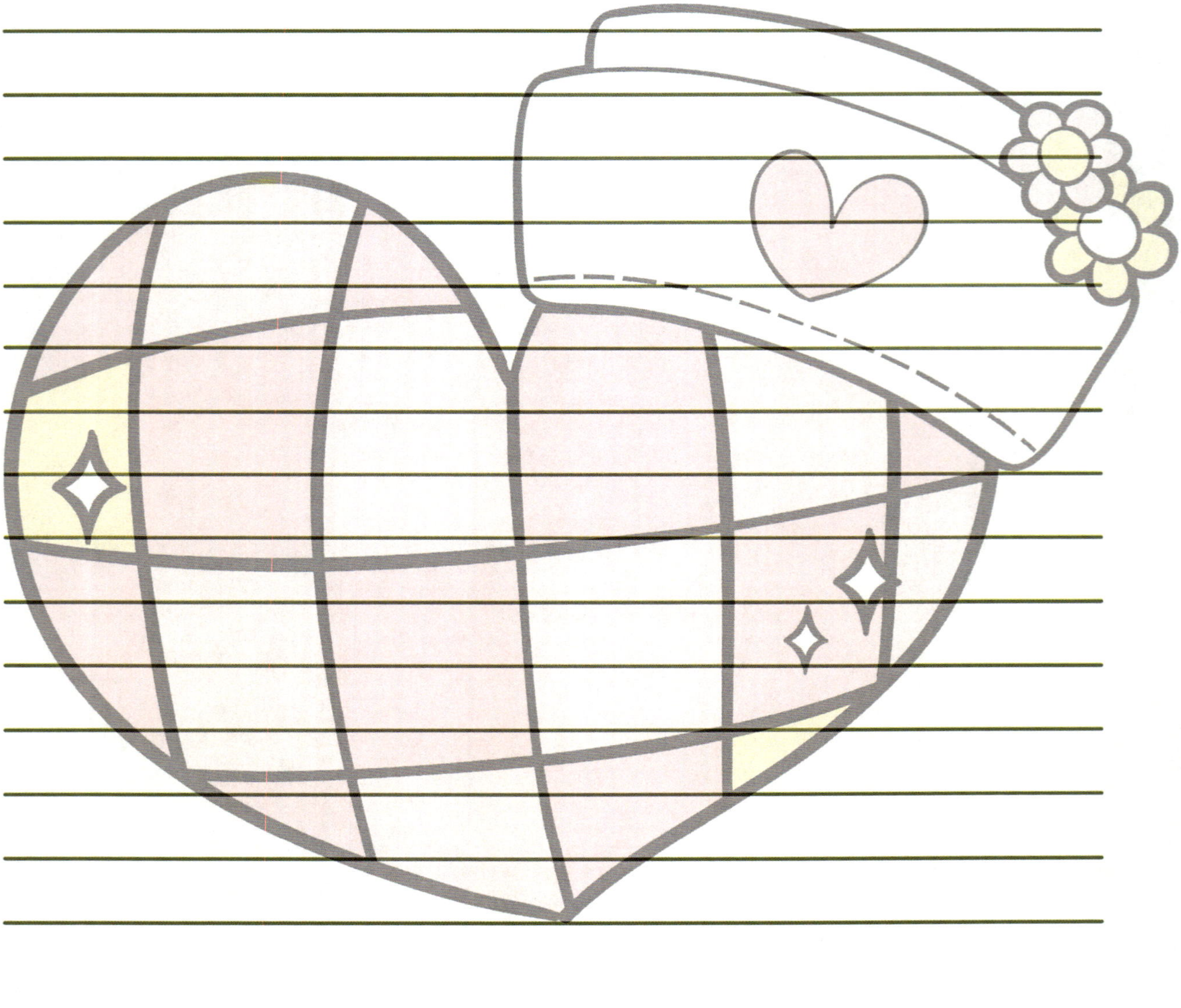

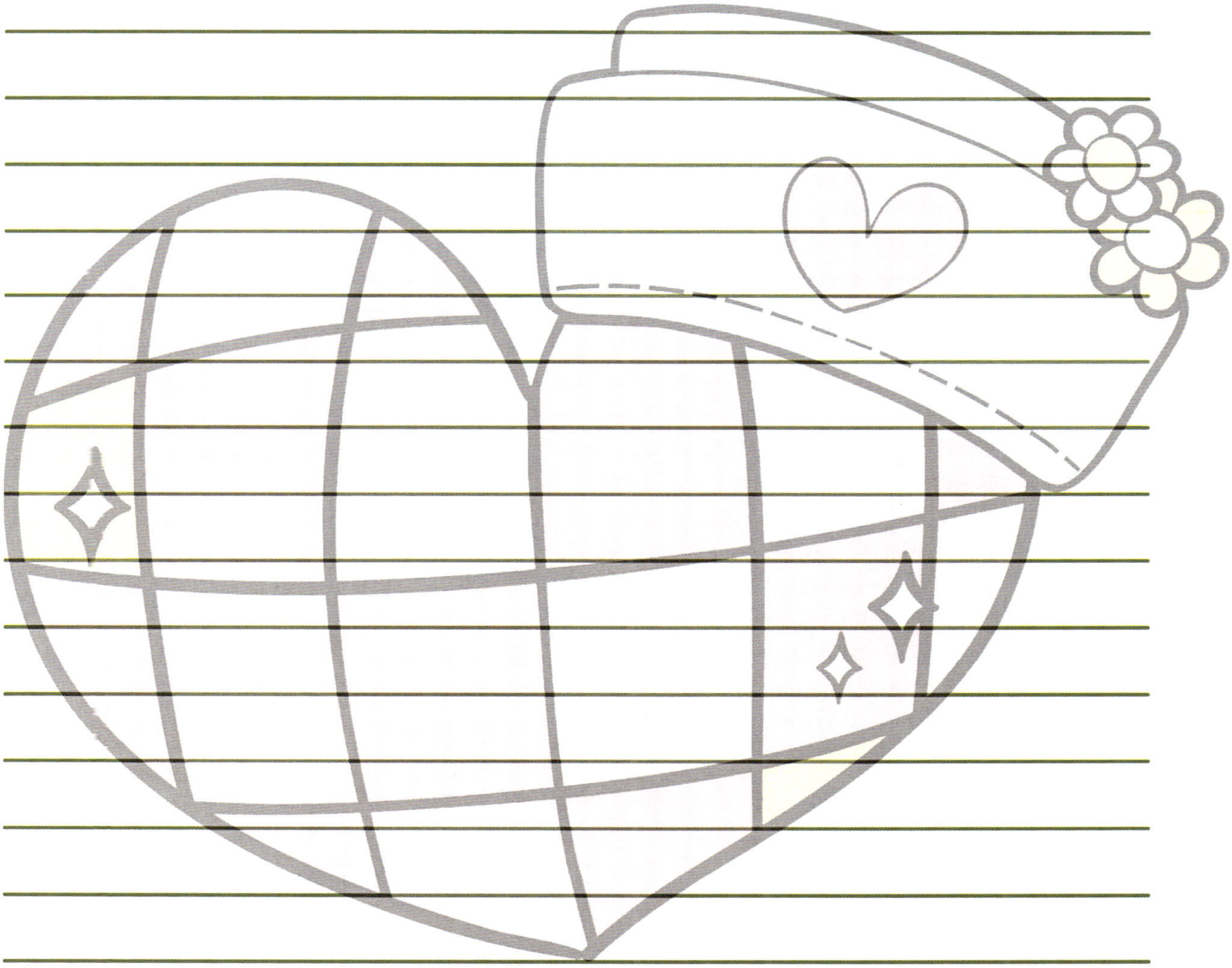

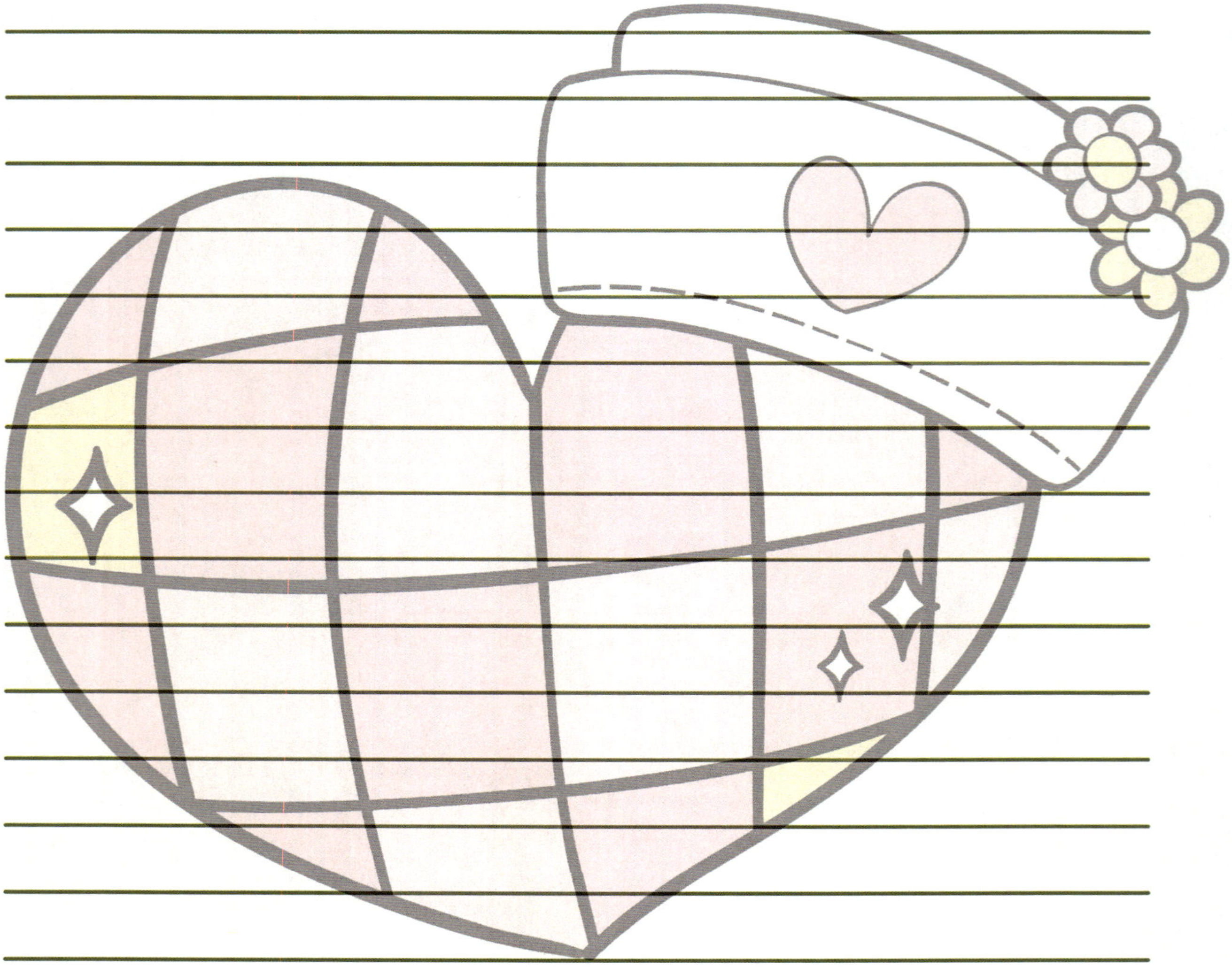

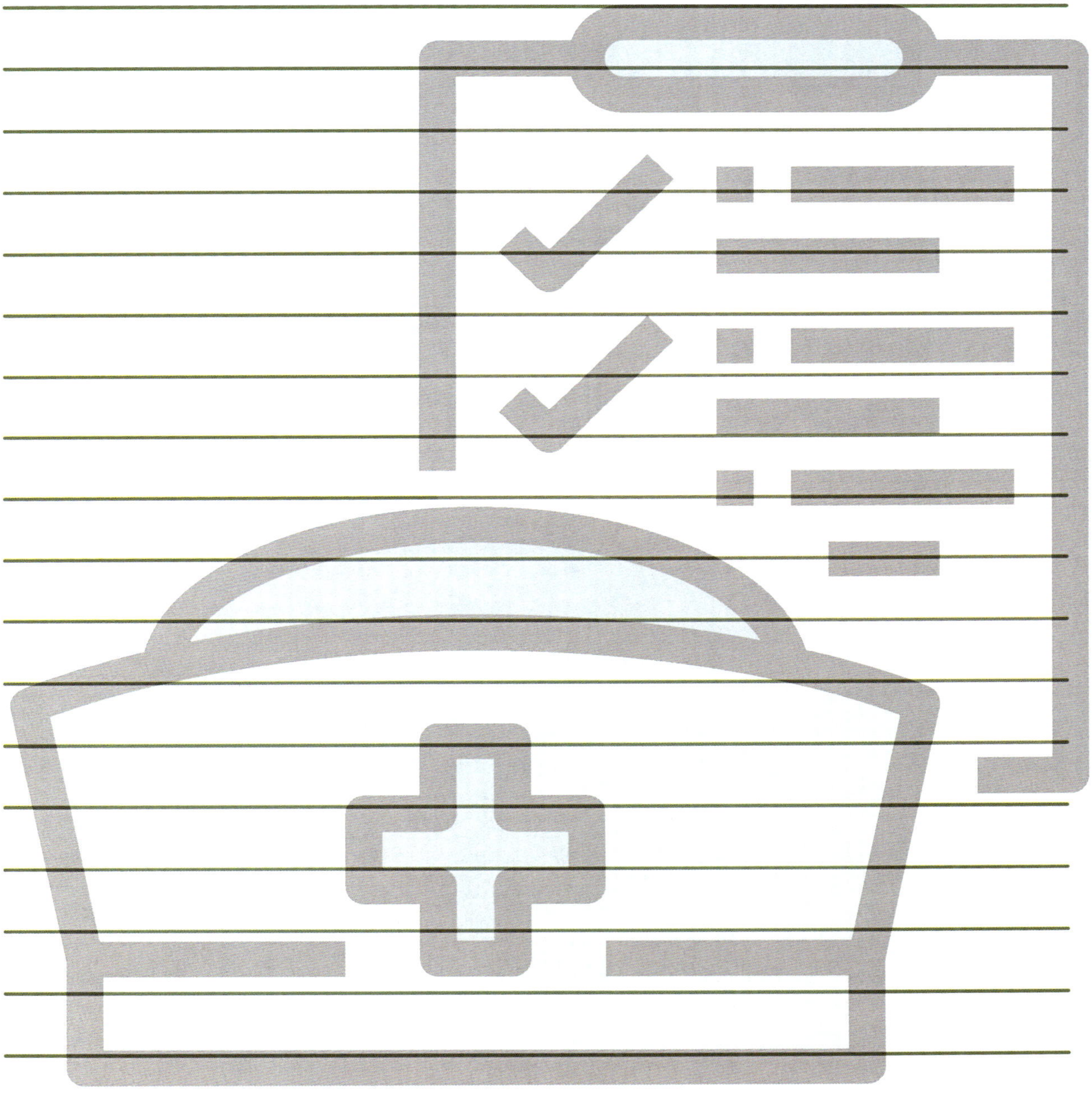

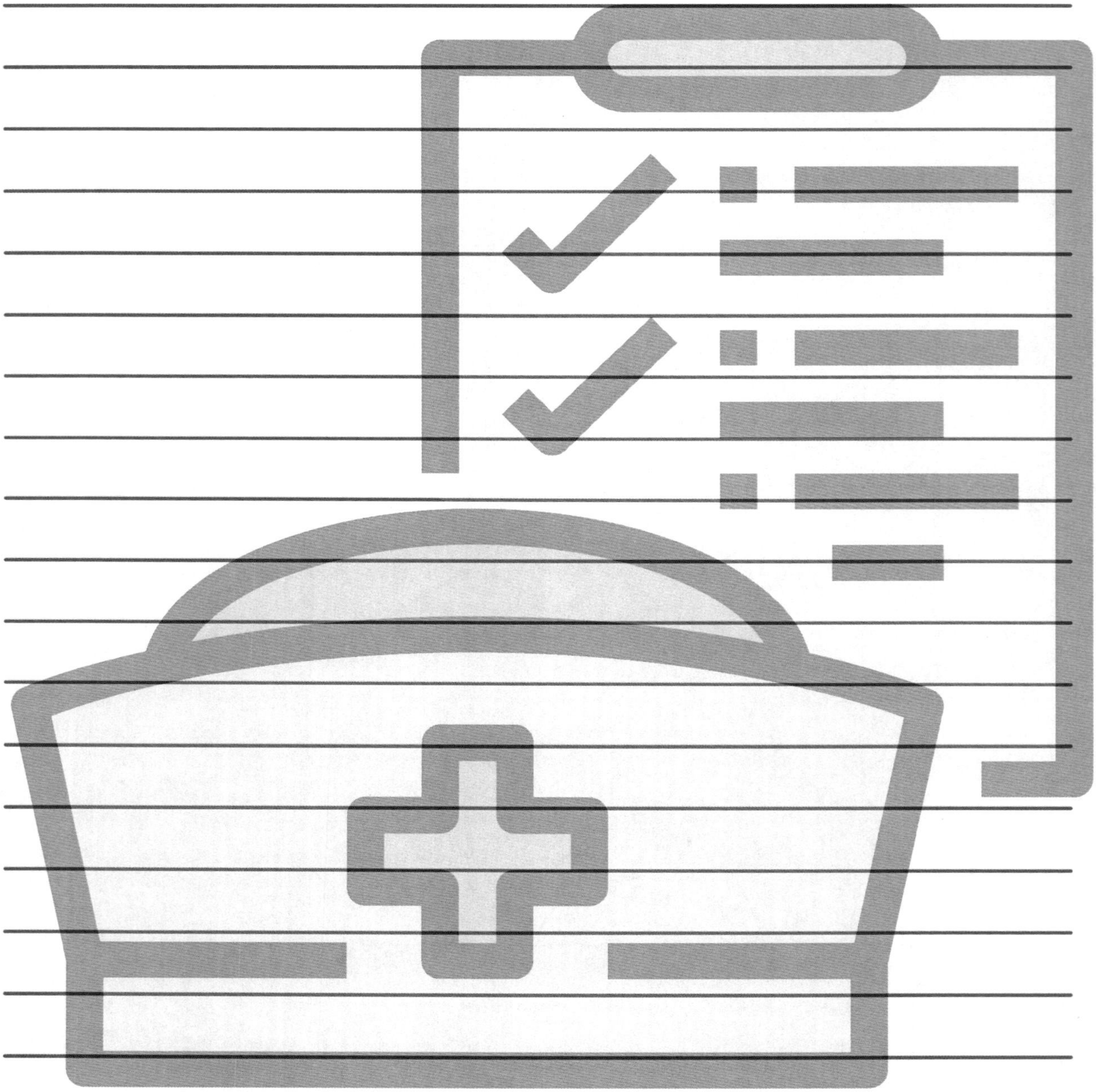

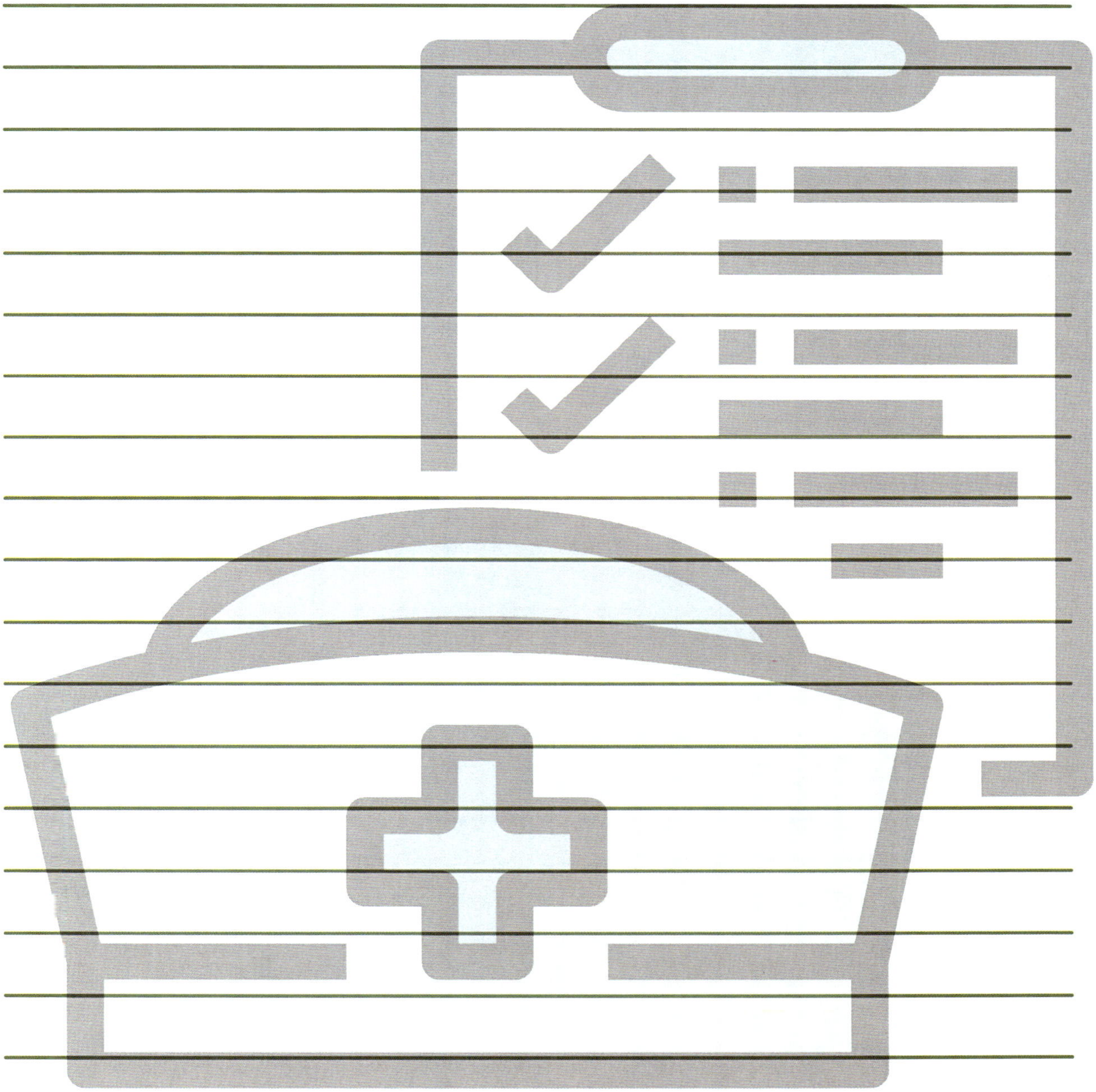

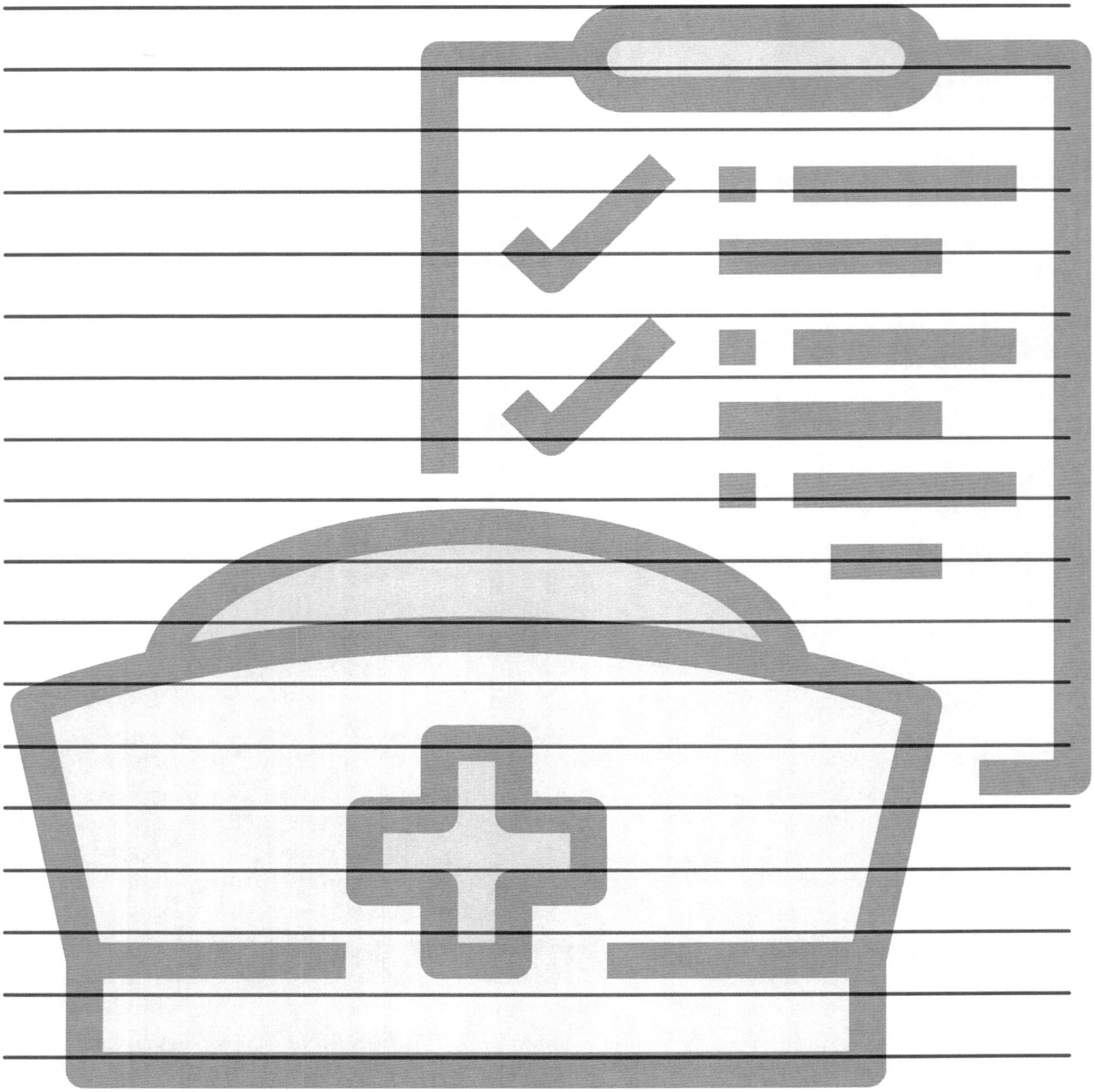

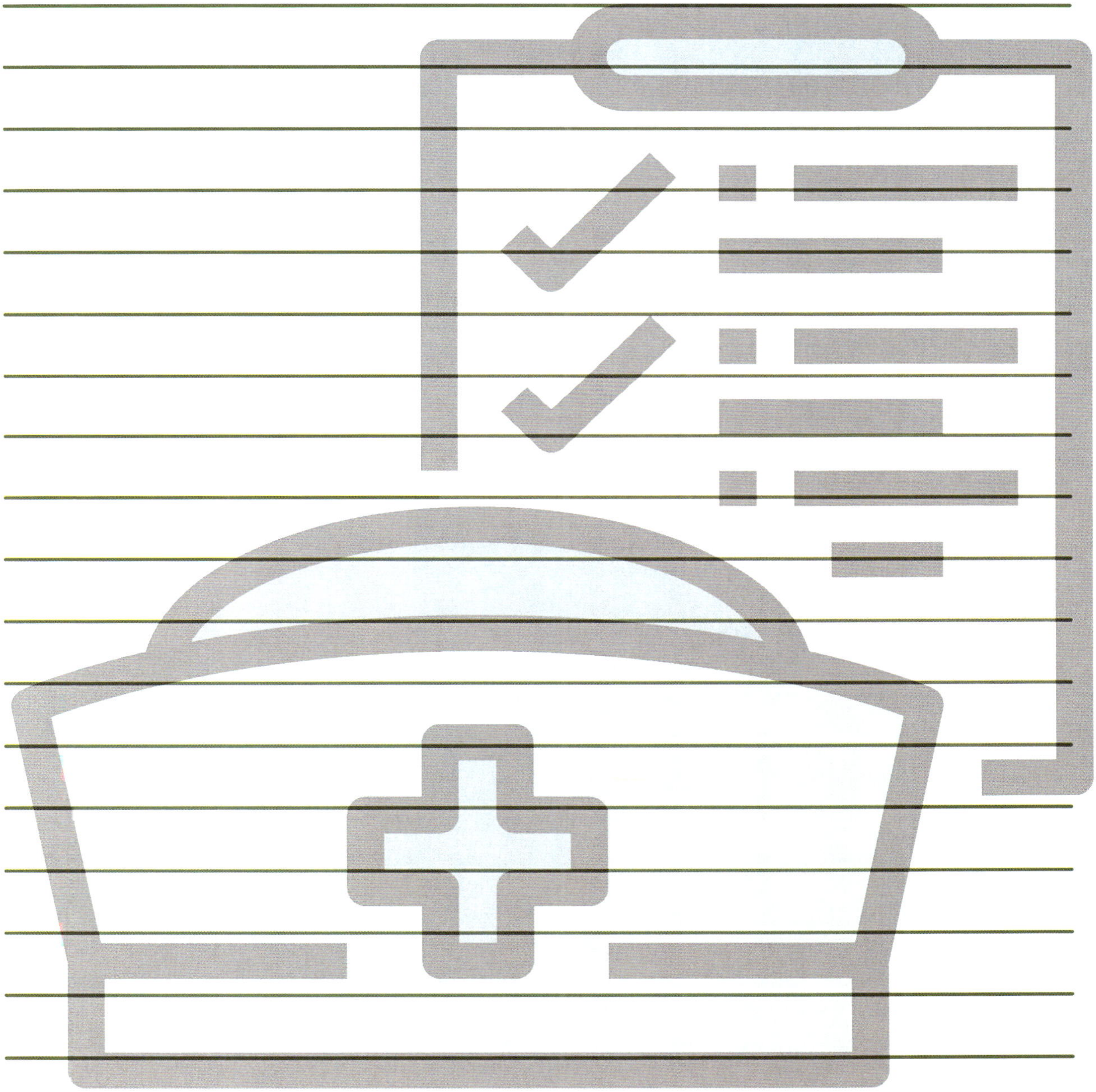

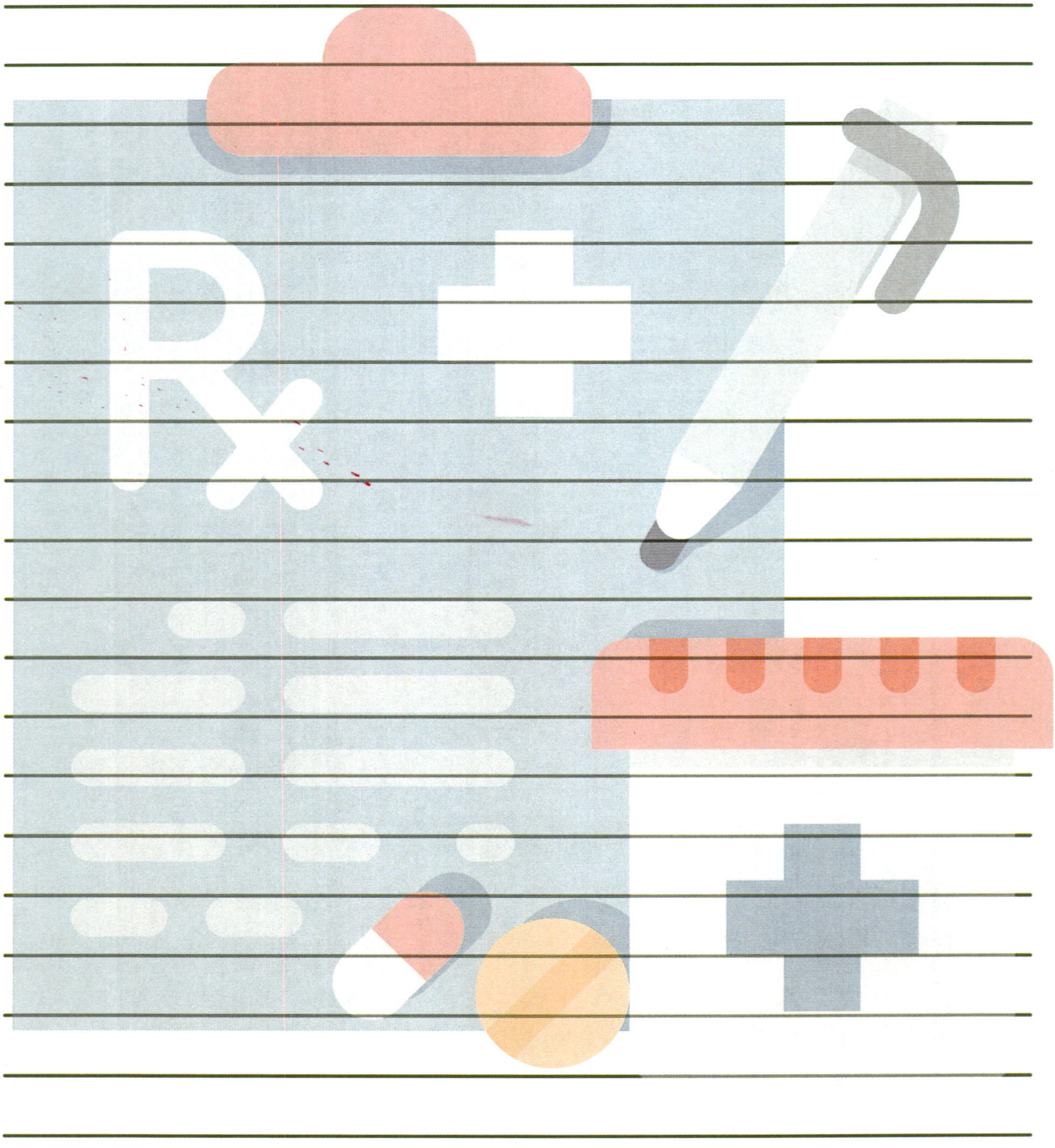
Rx

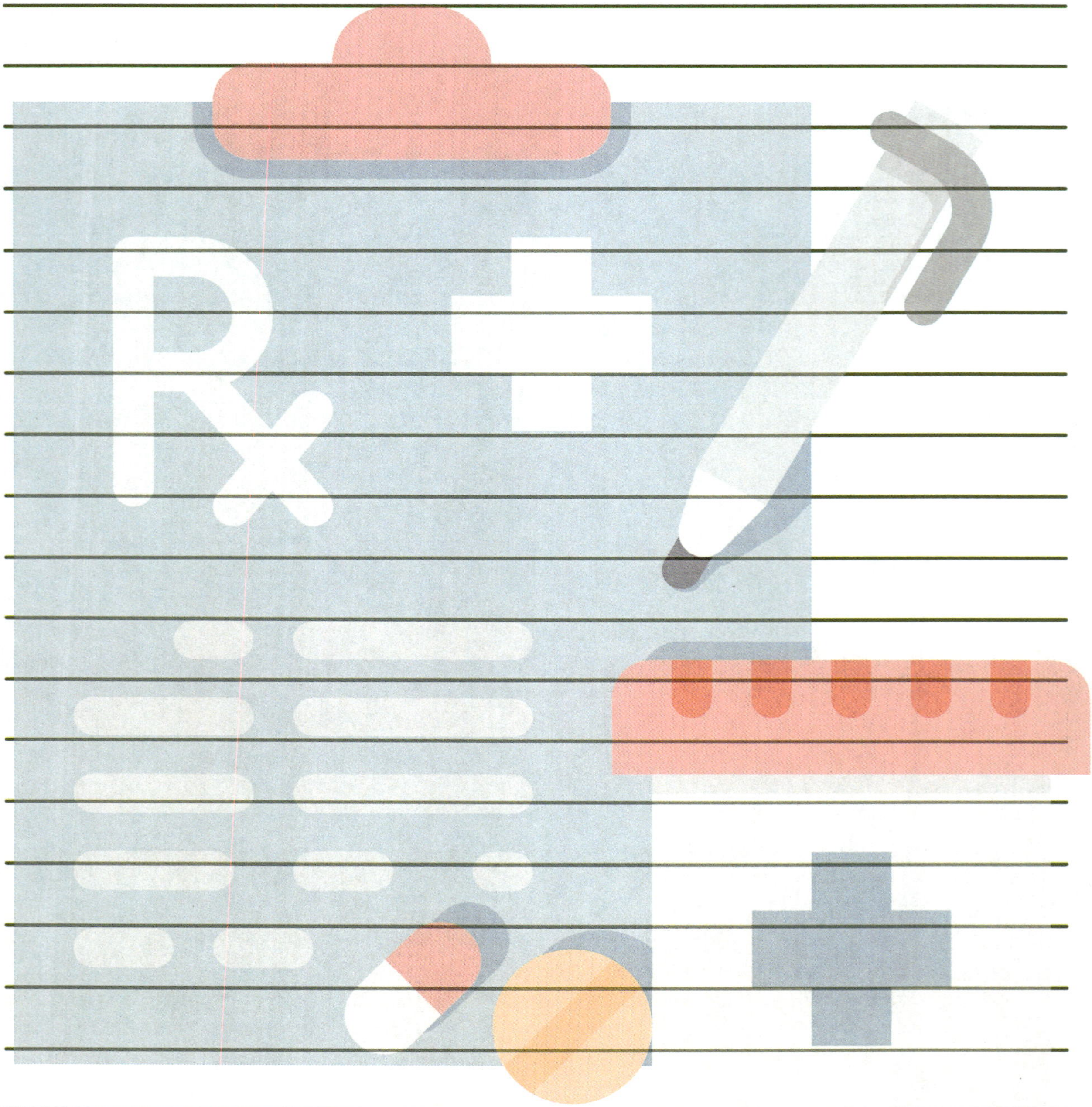

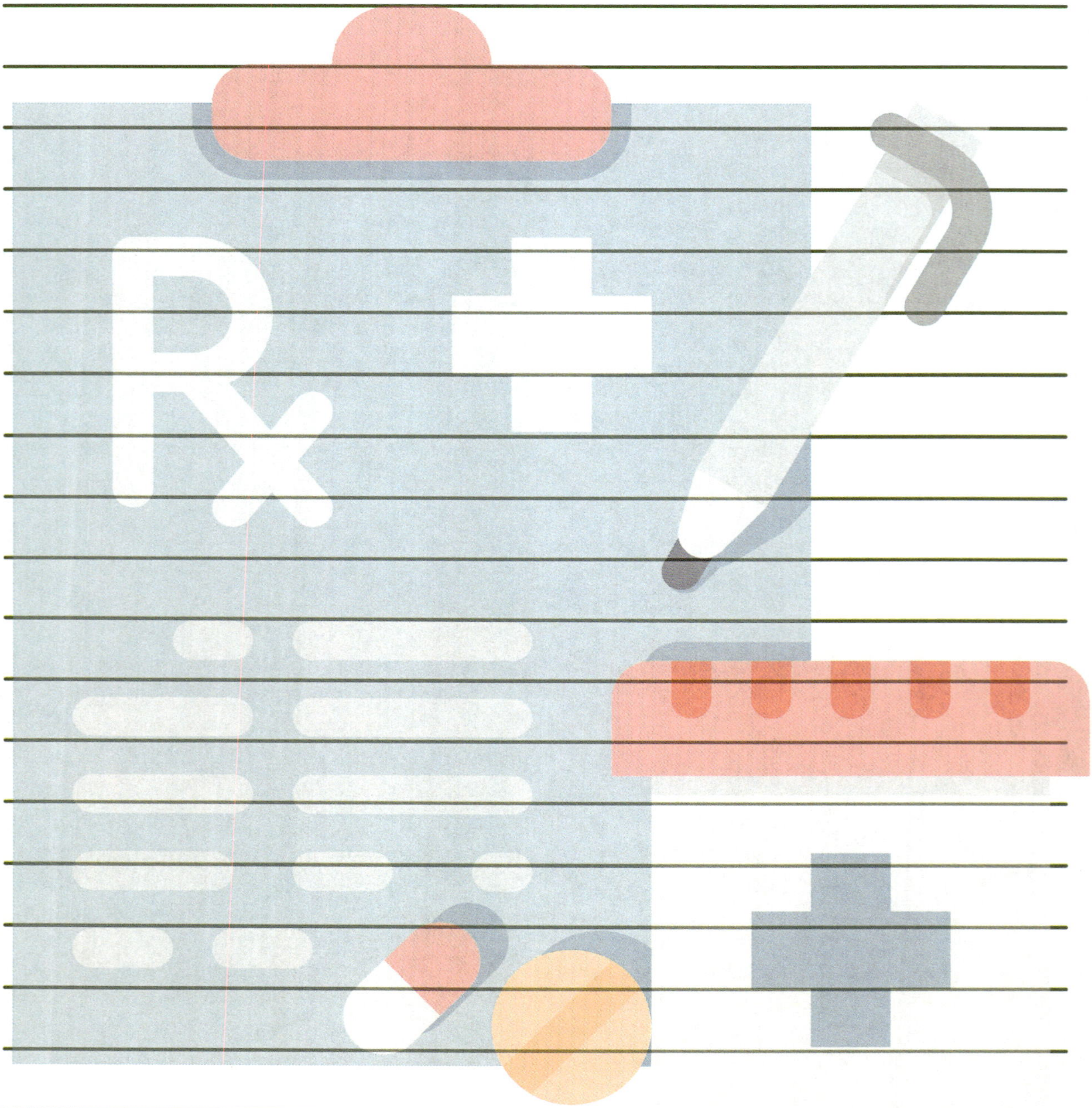

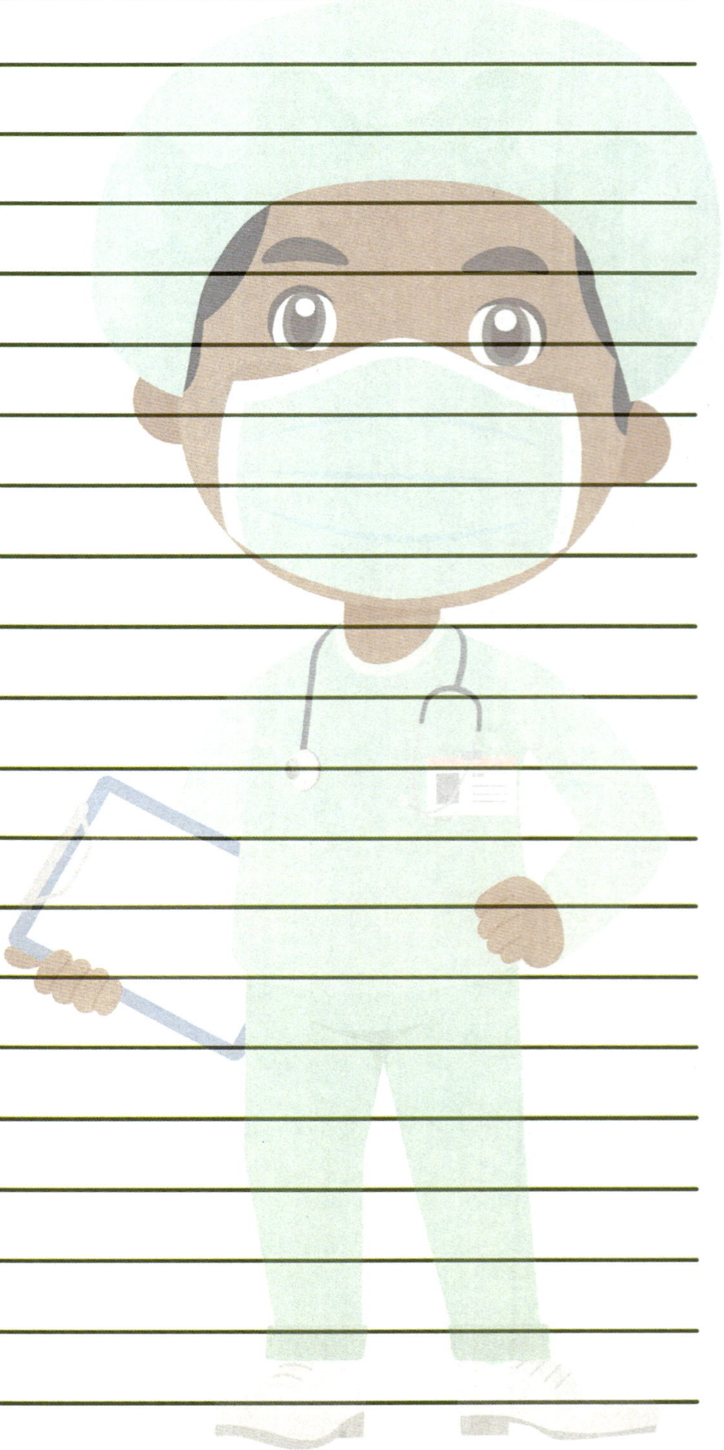

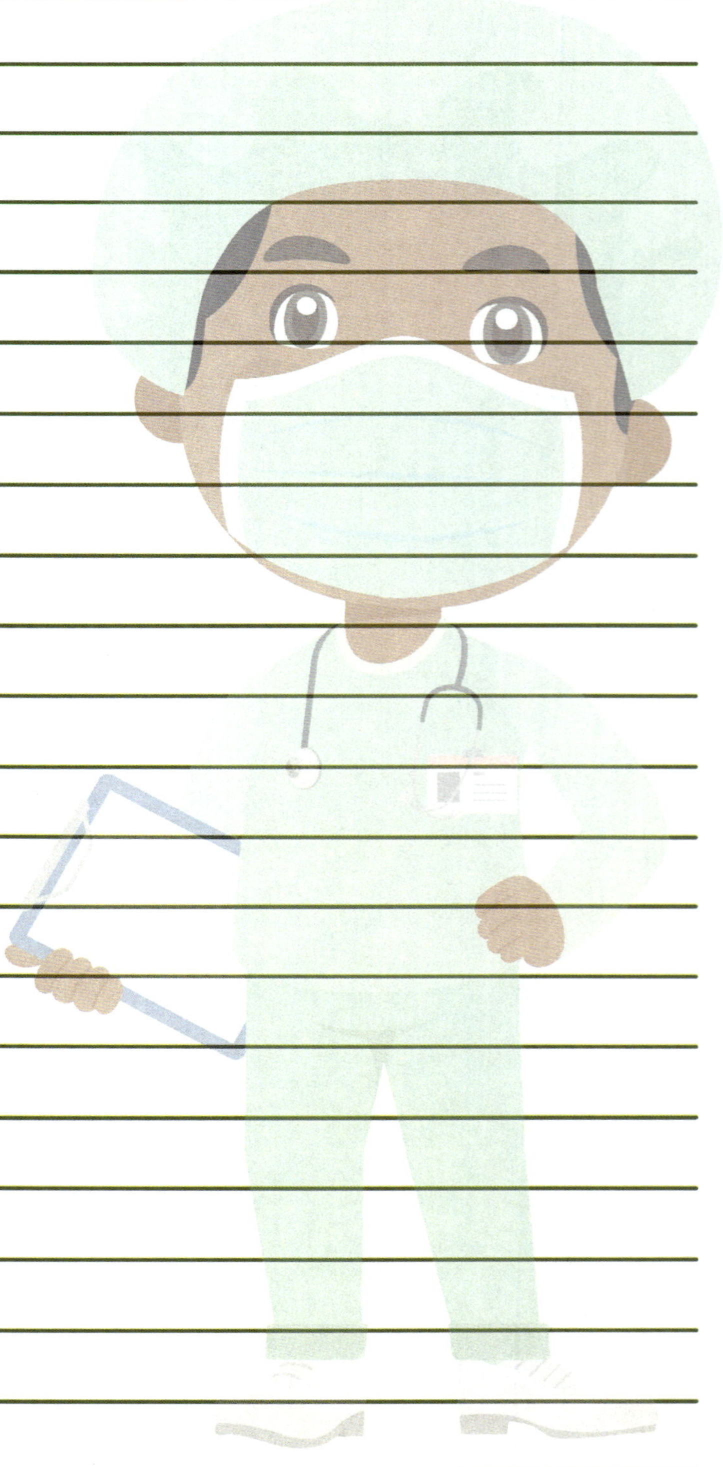

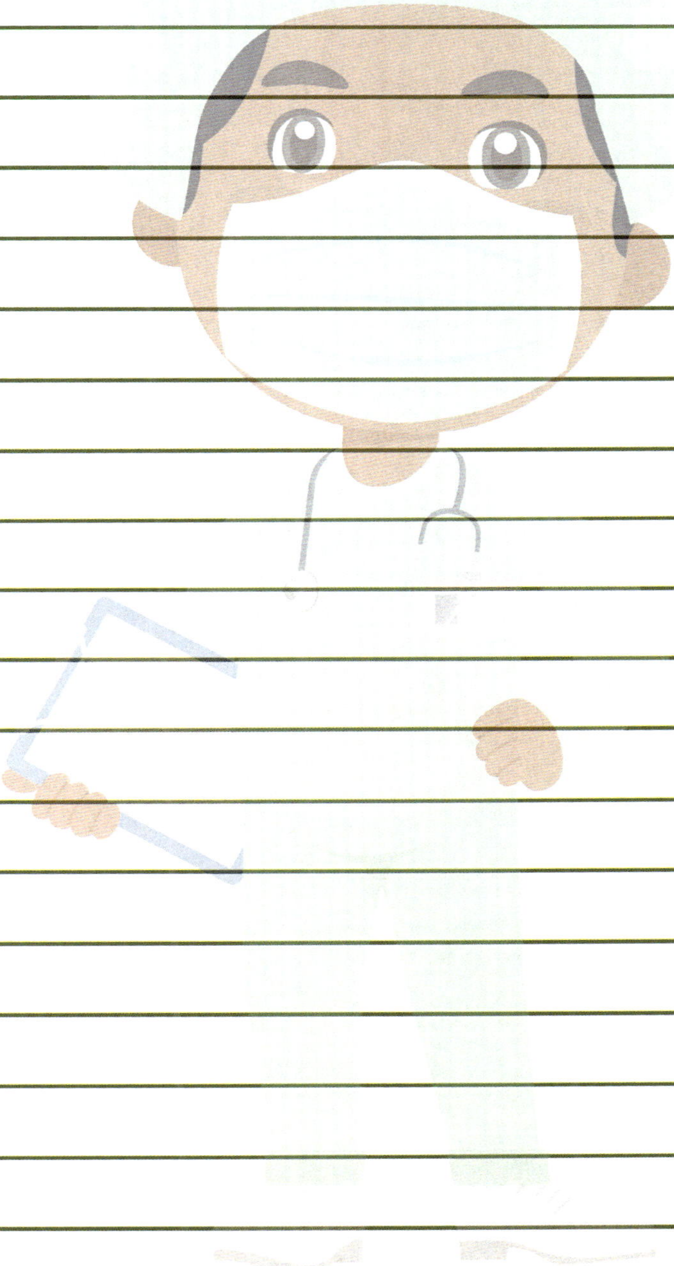

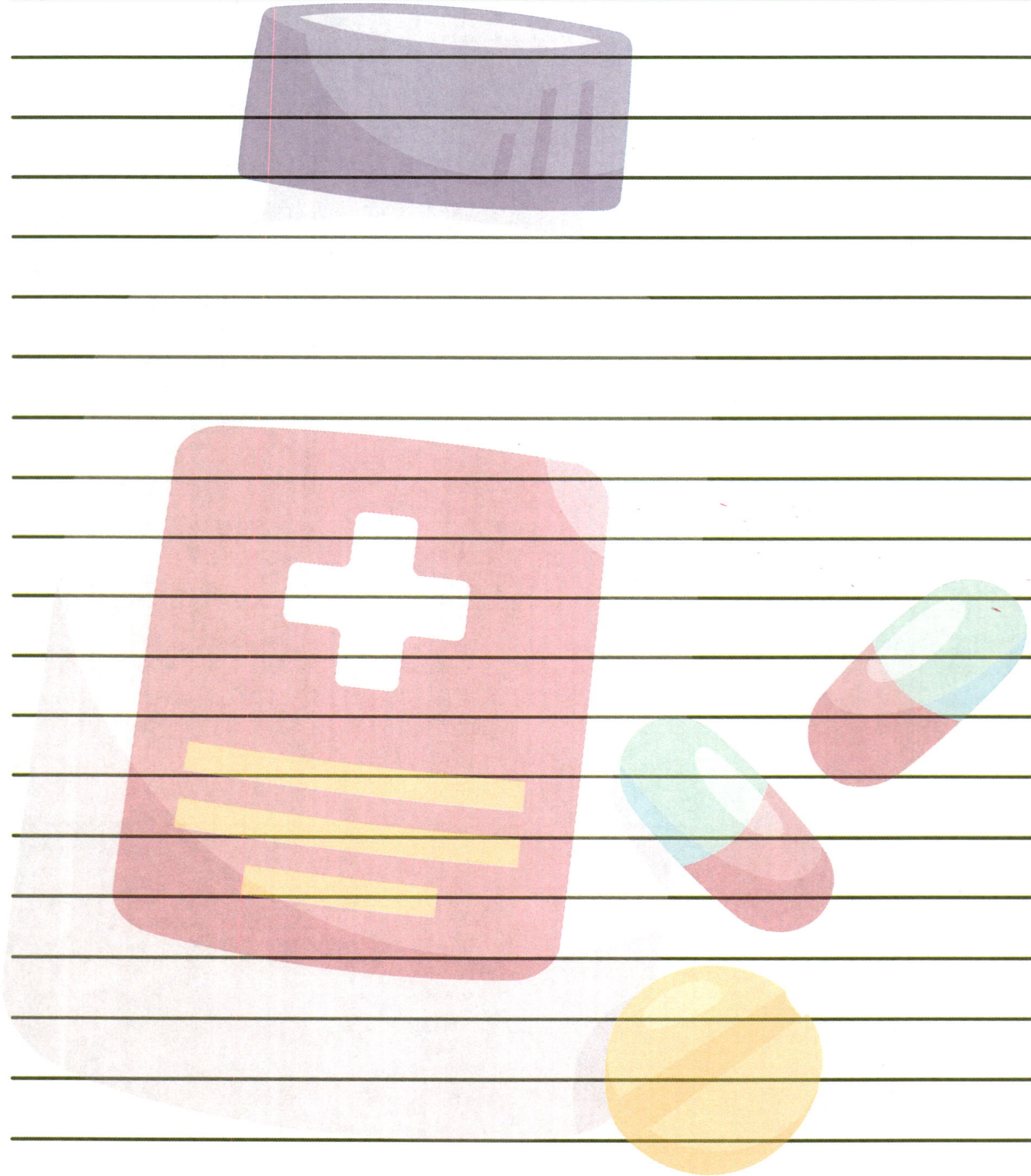

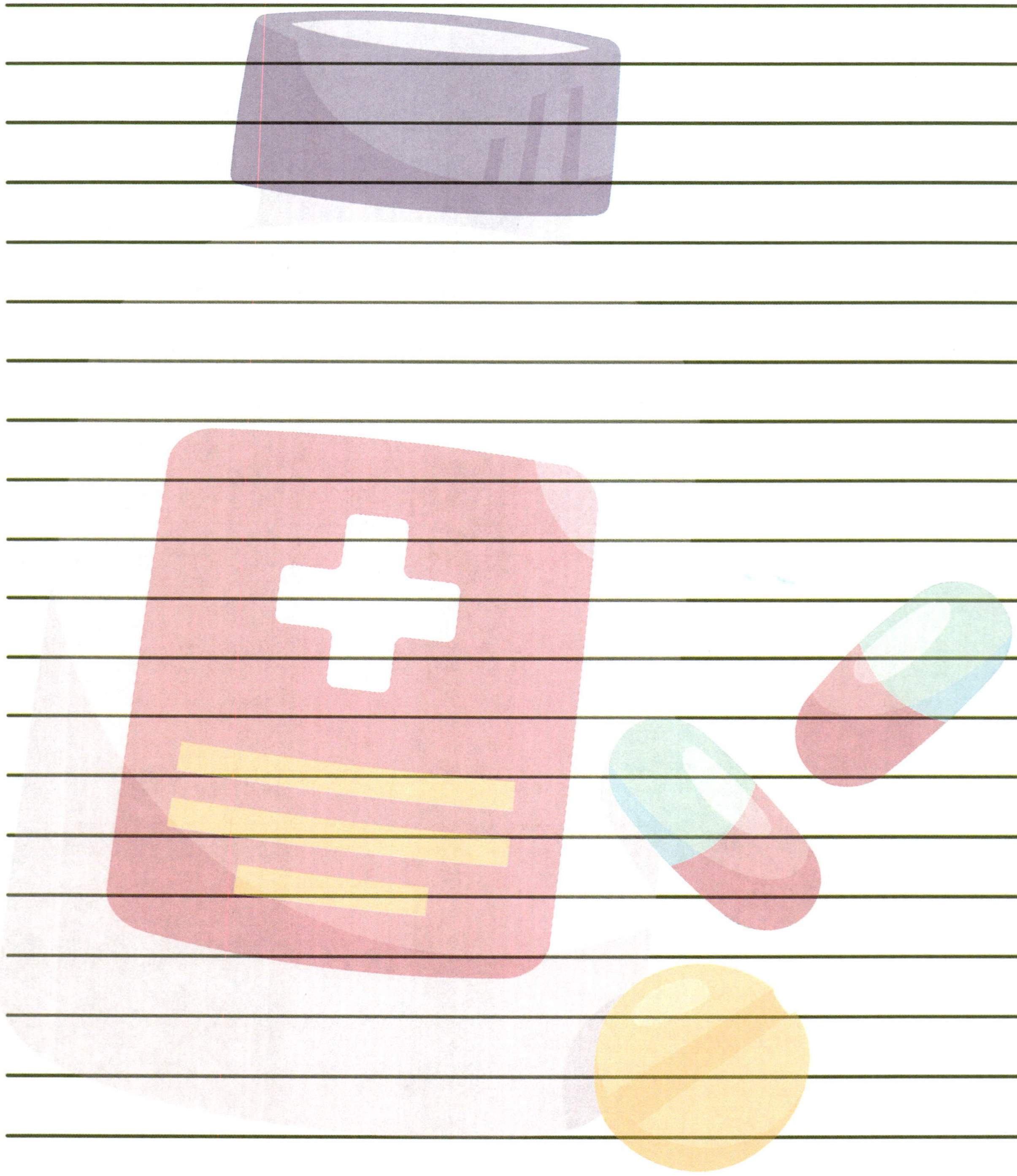

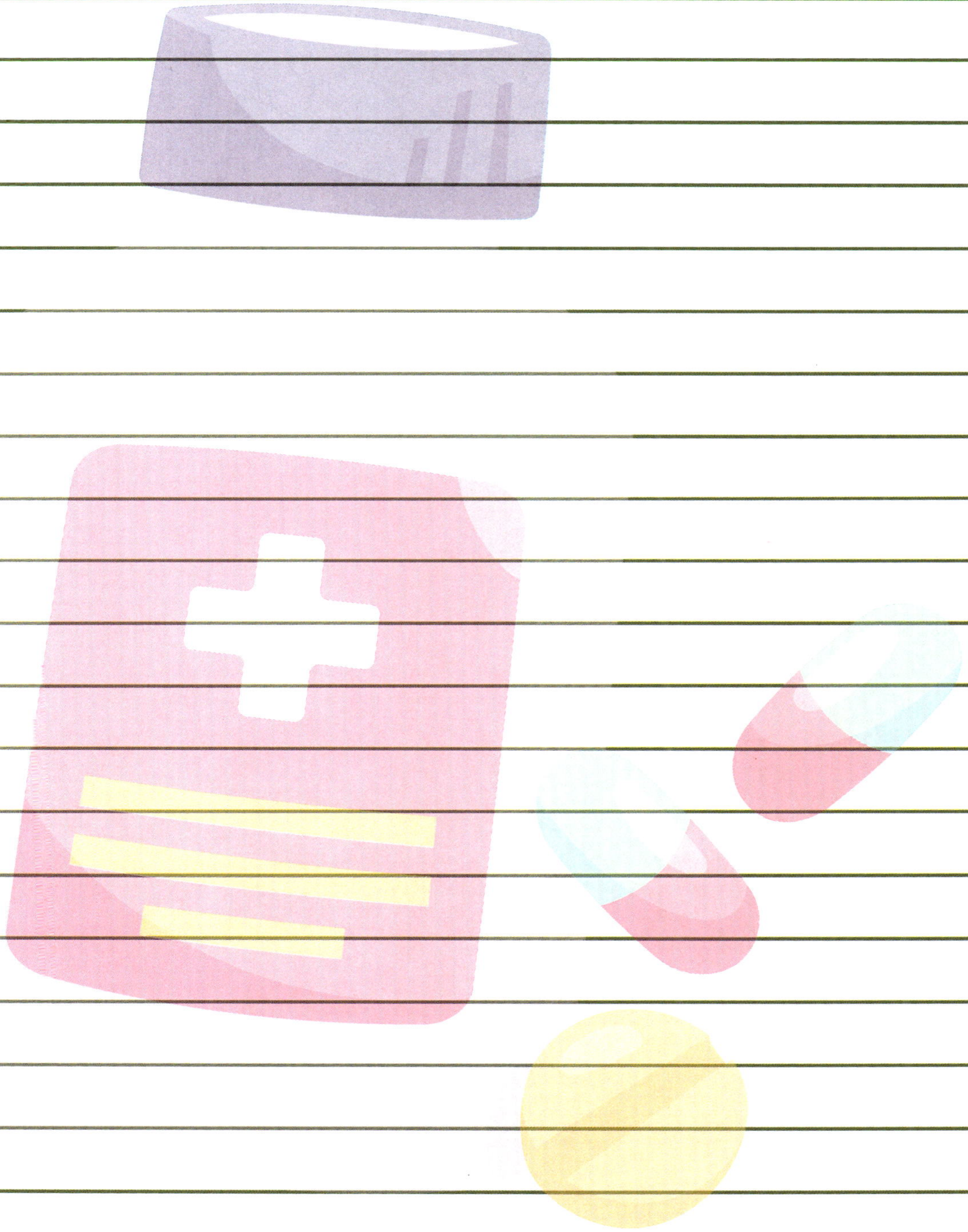

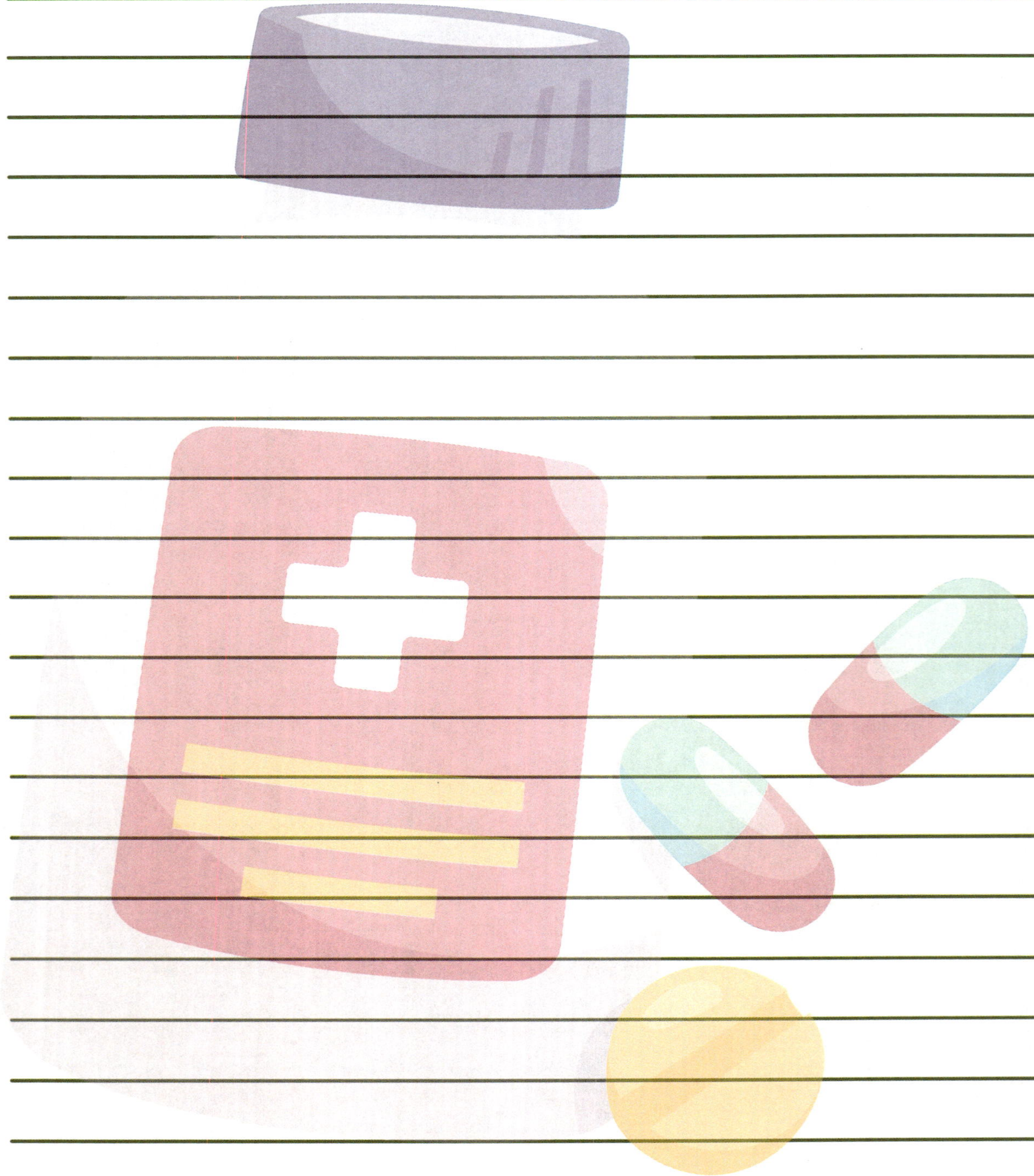

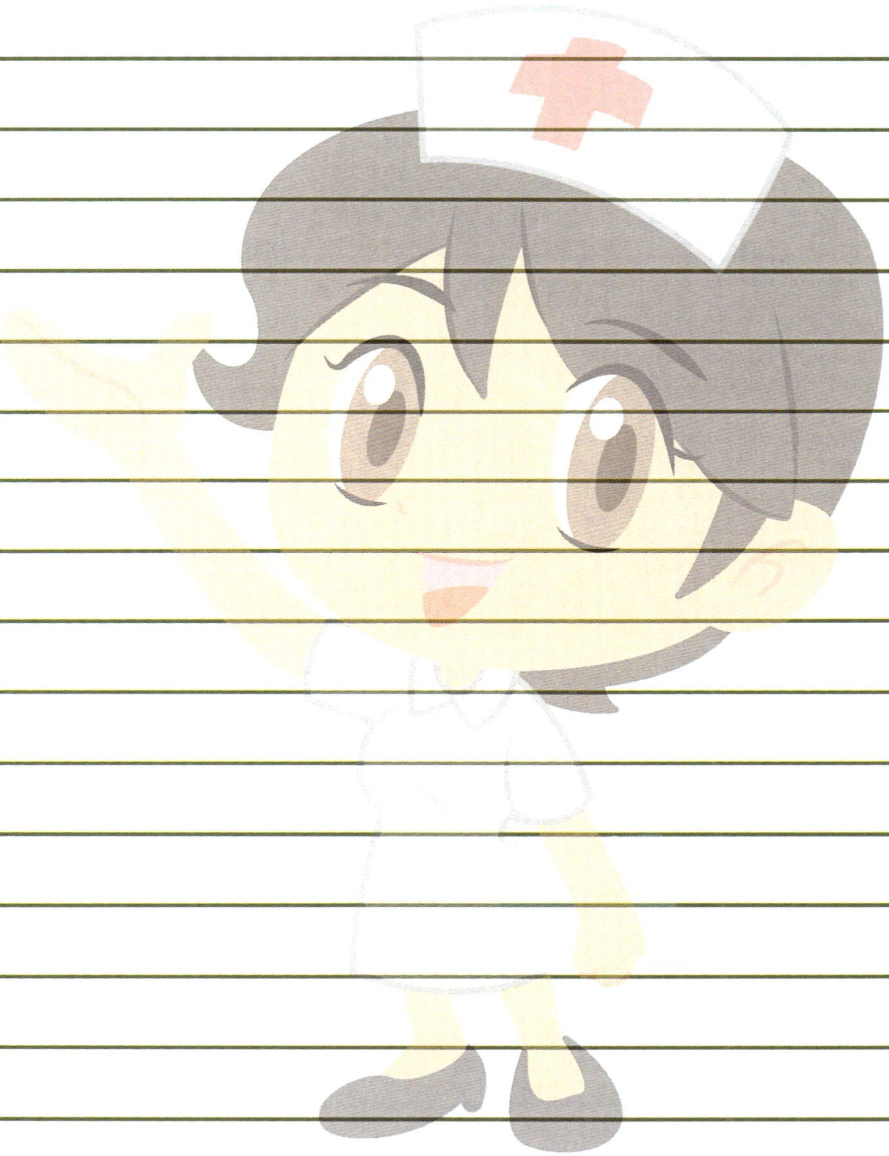

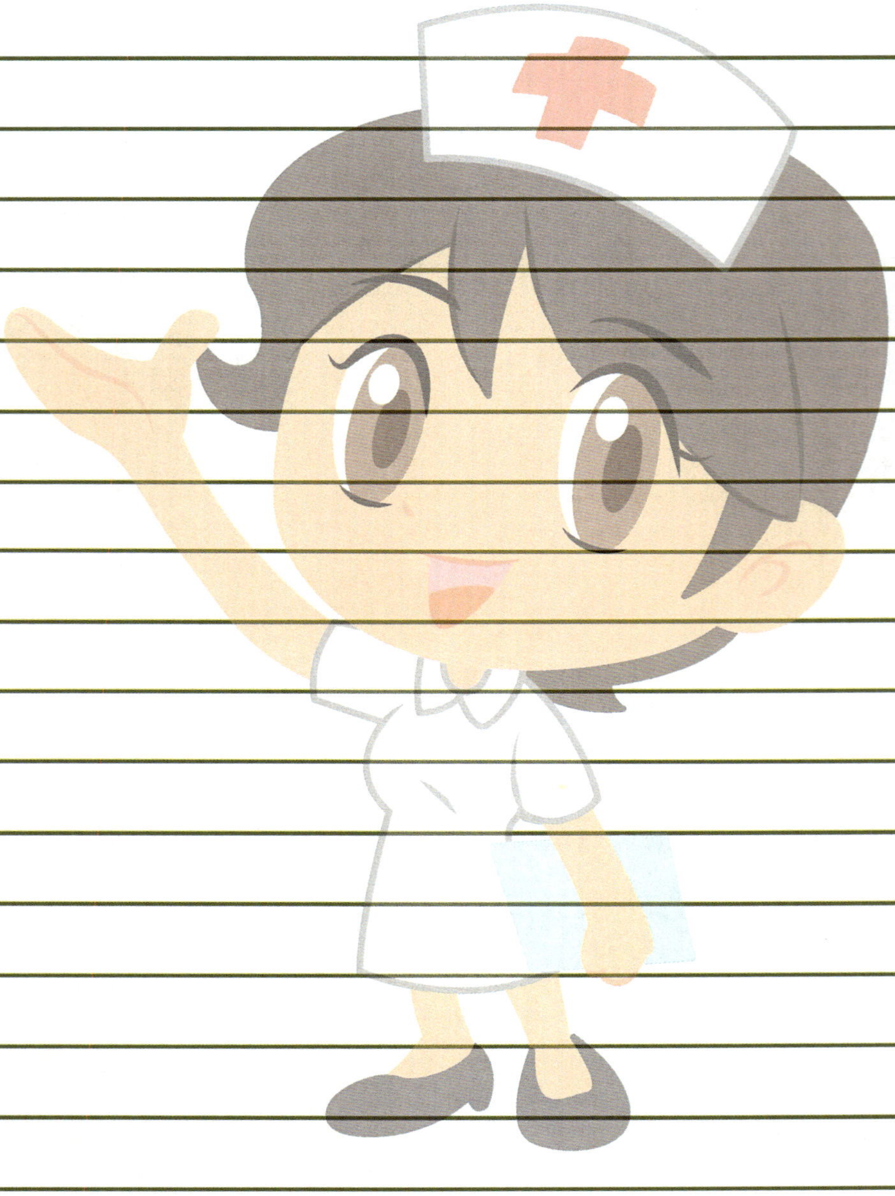

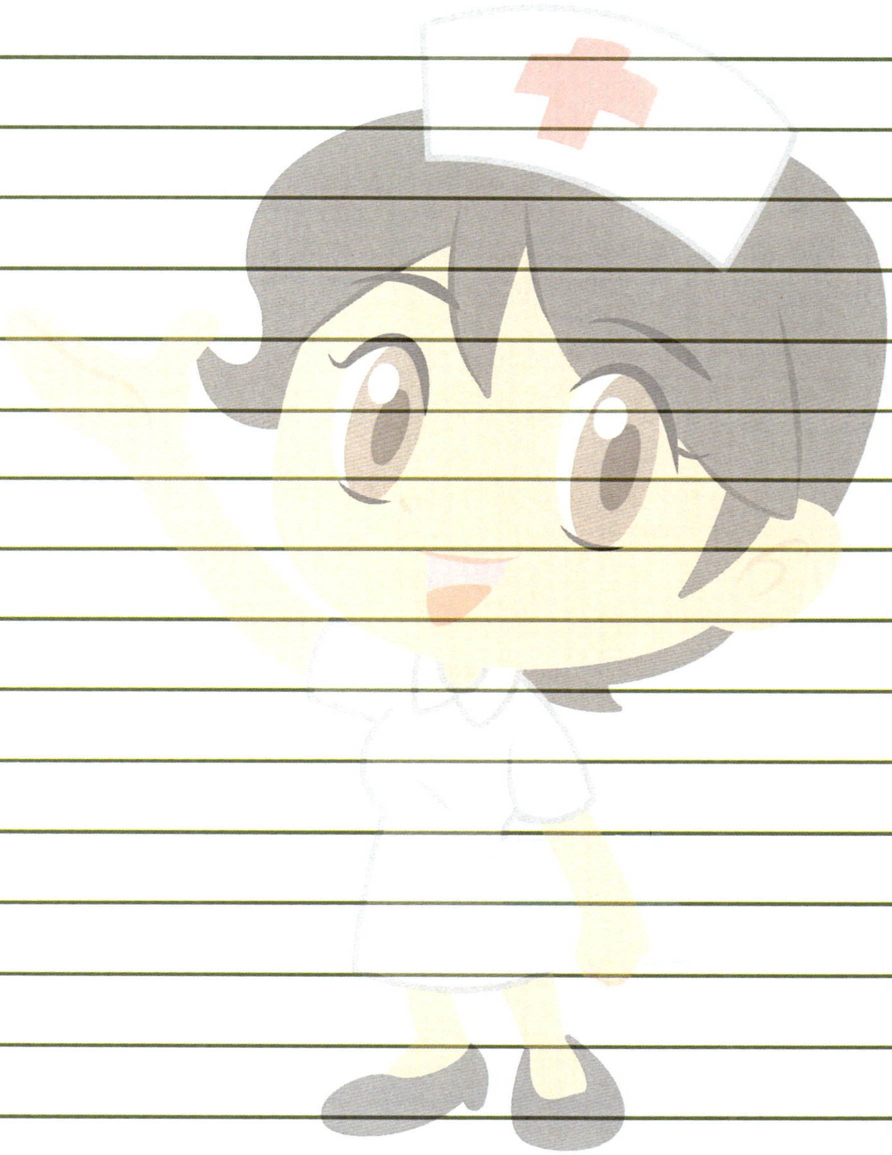

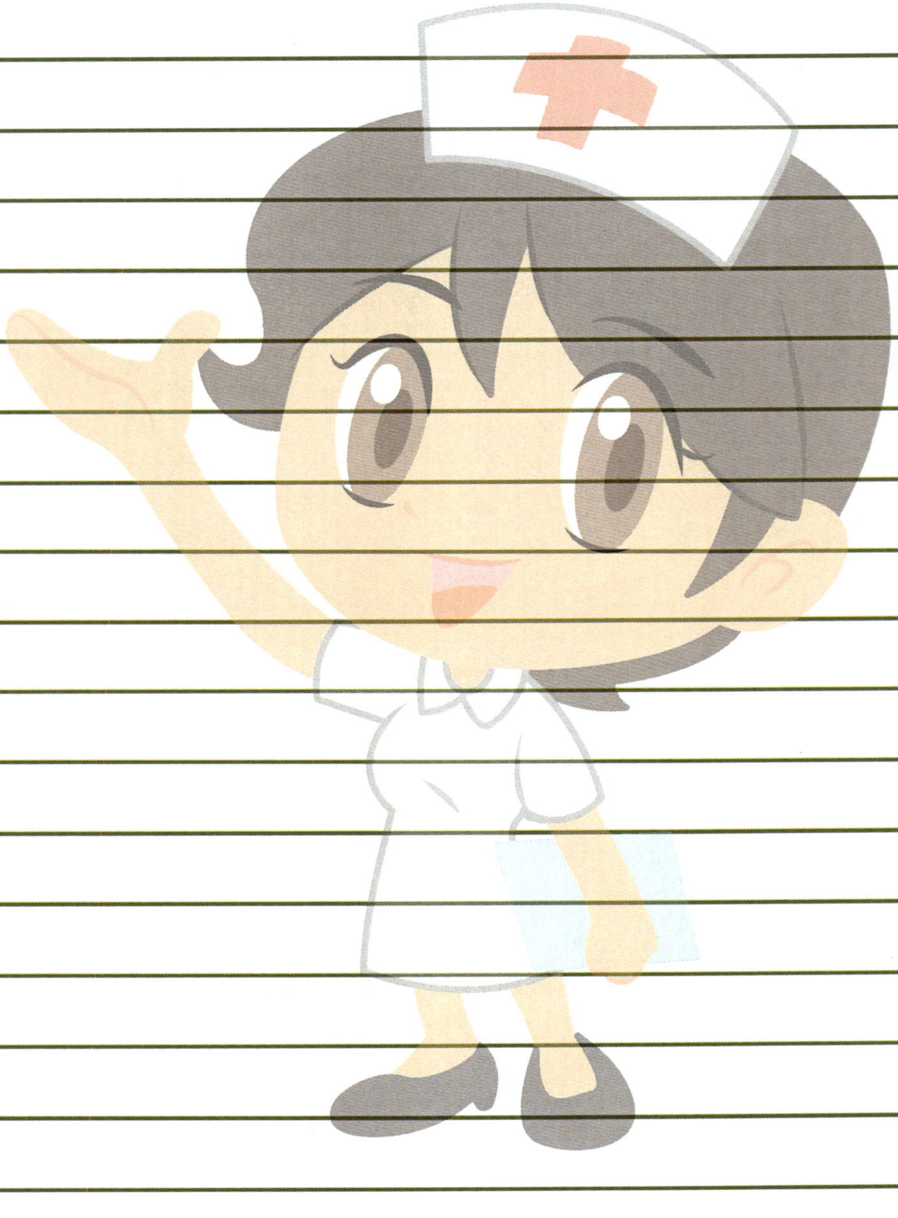

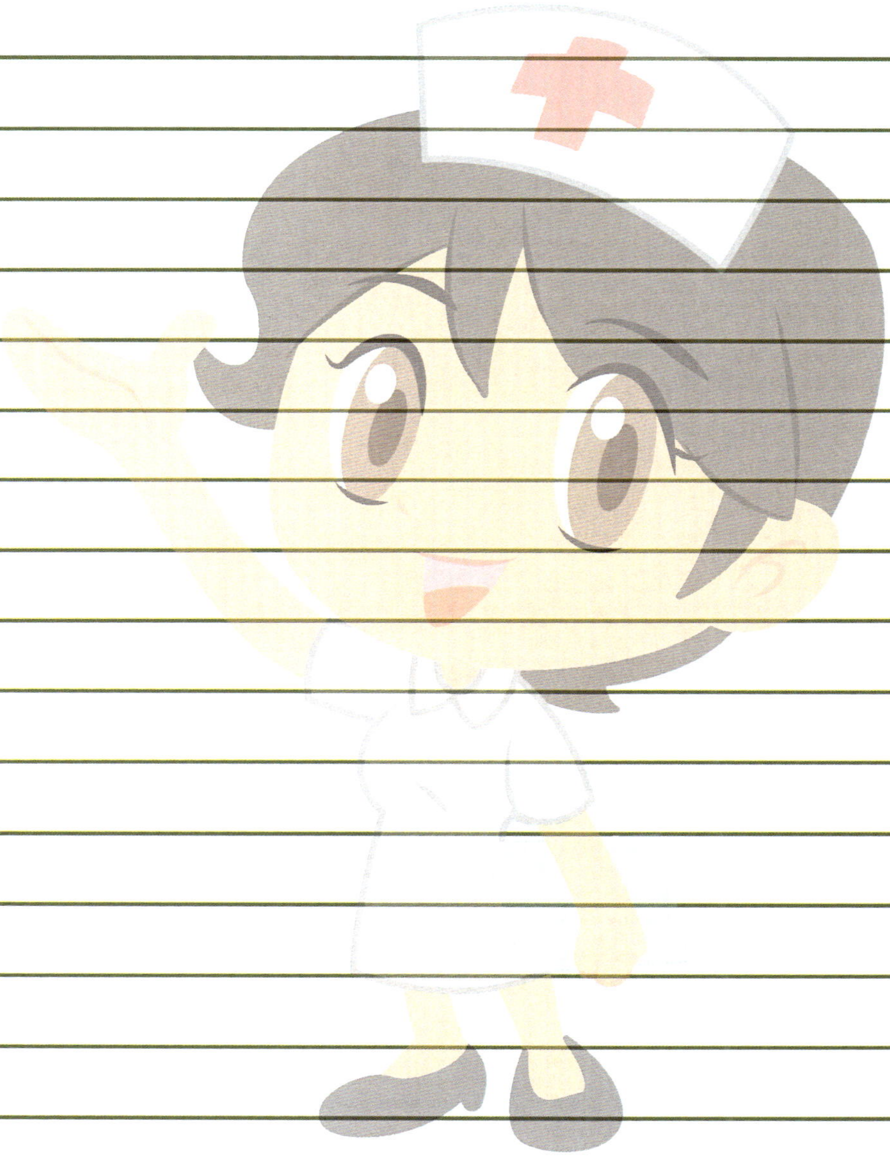

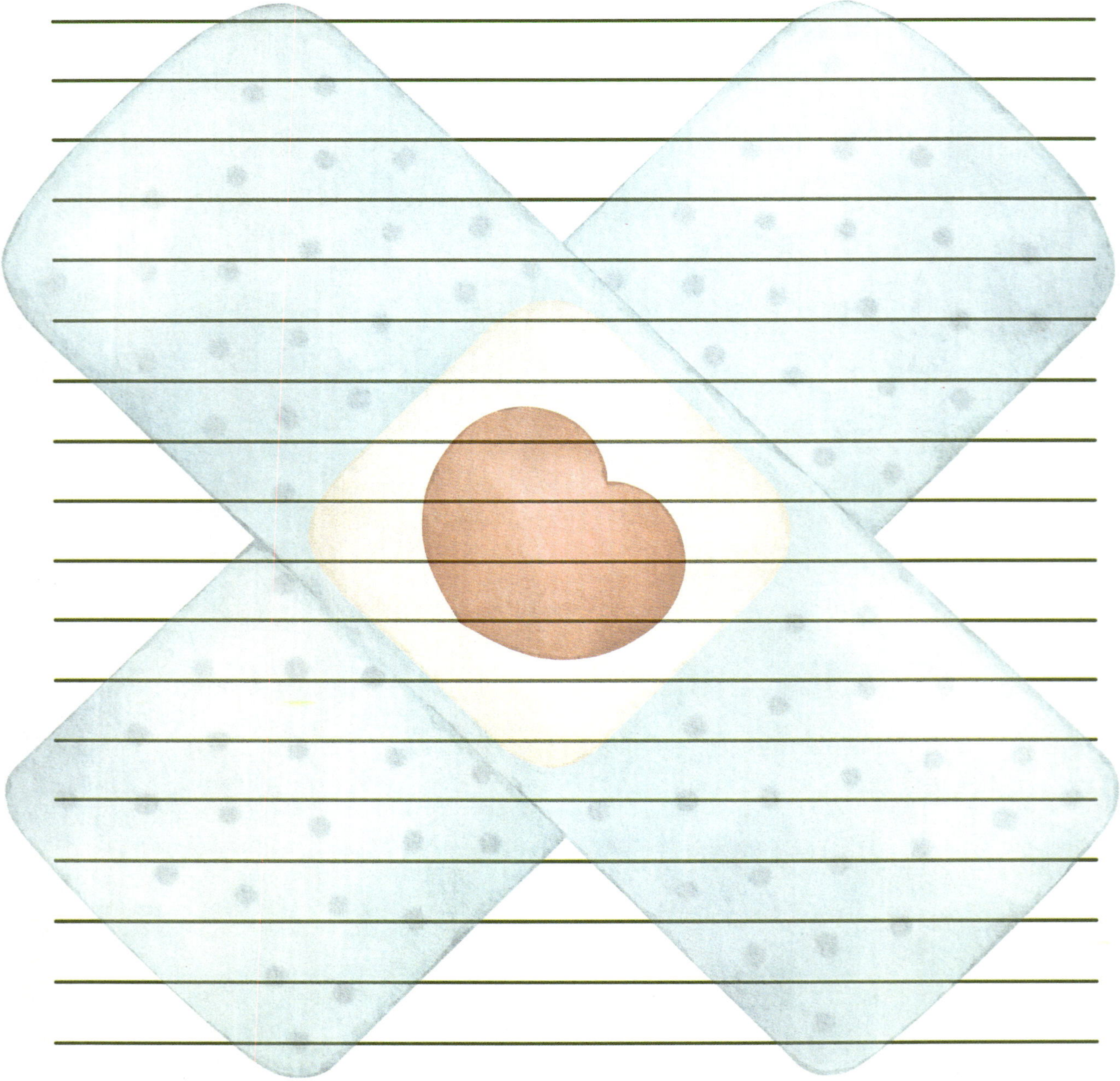

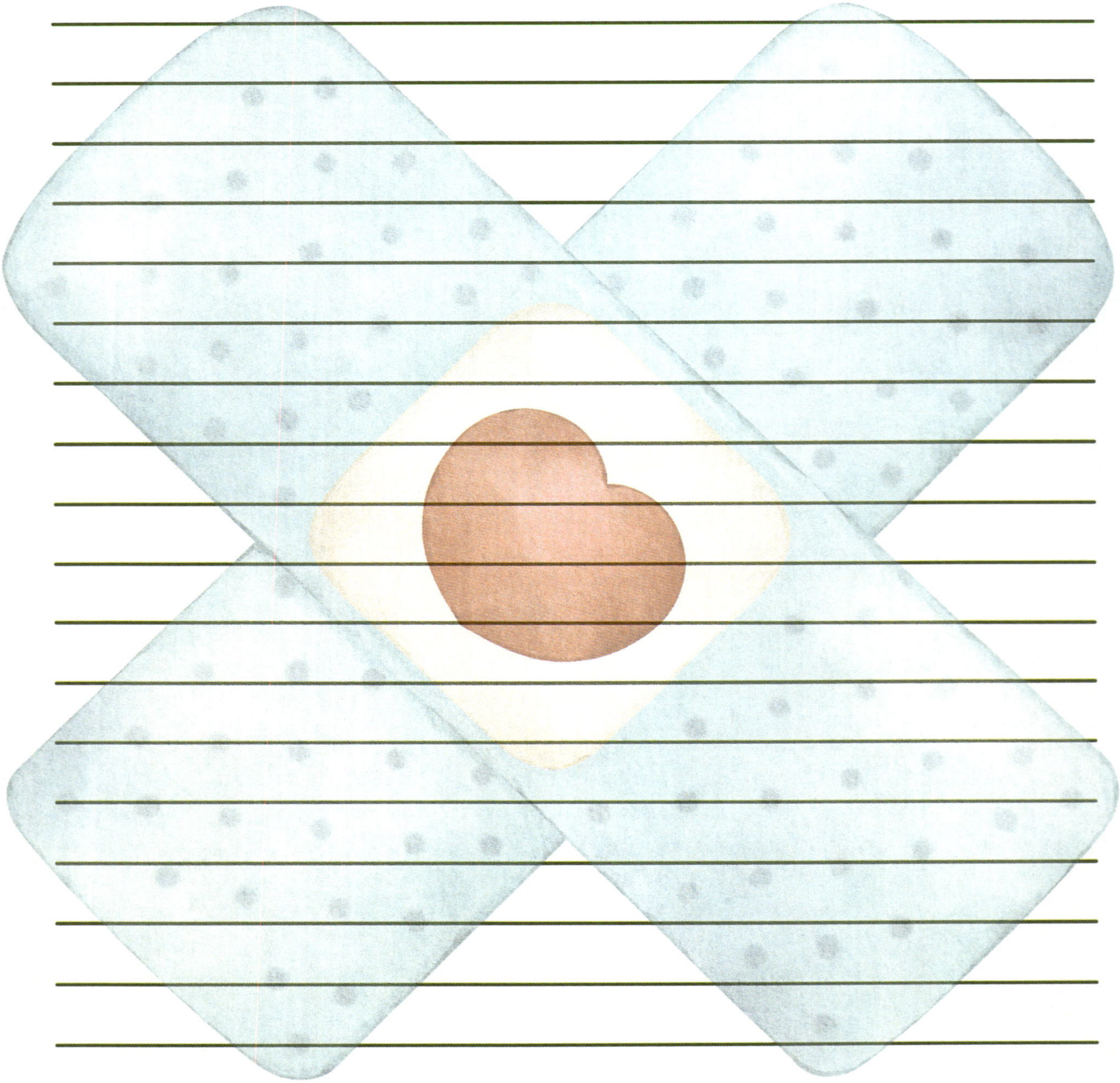

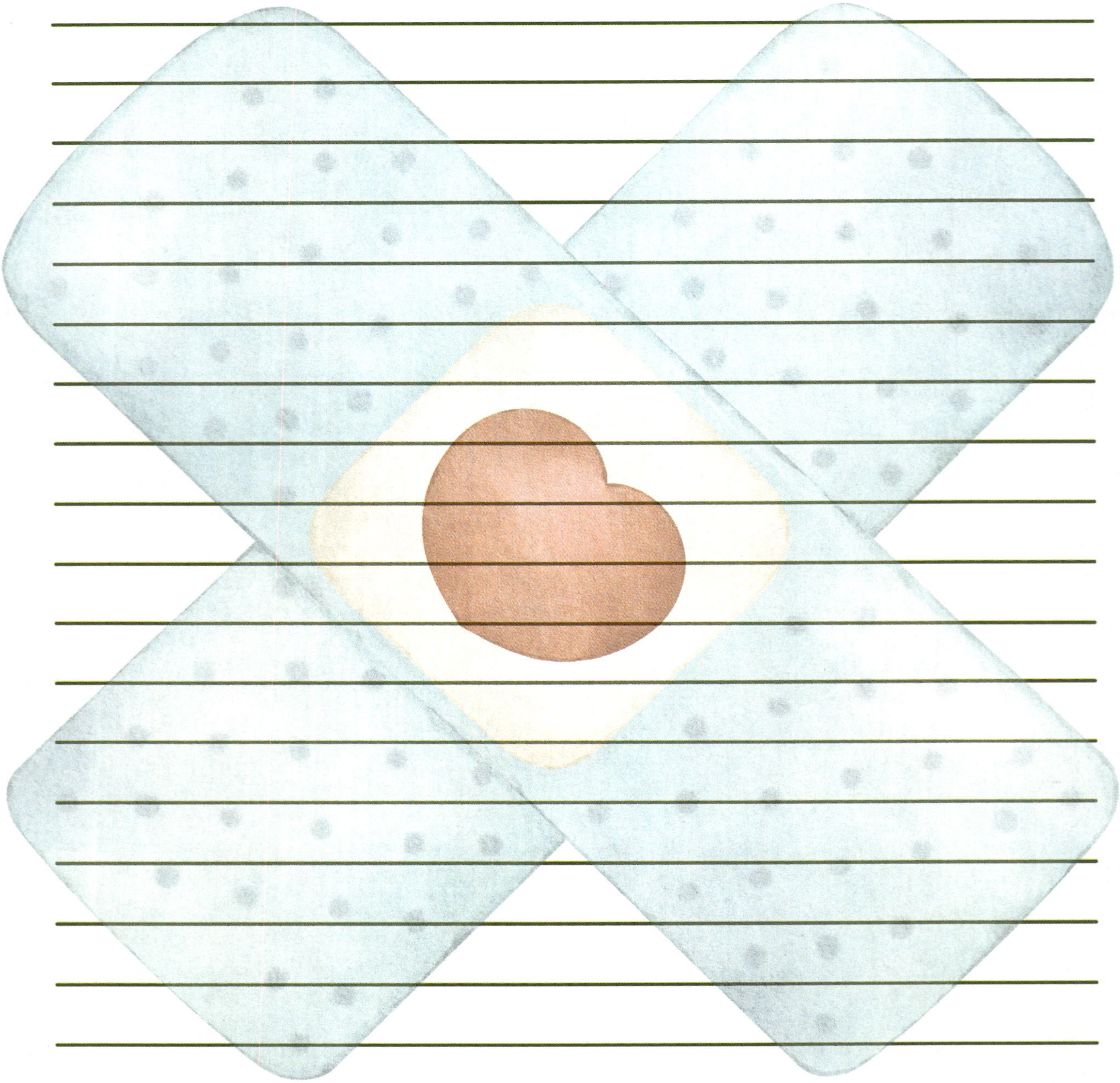

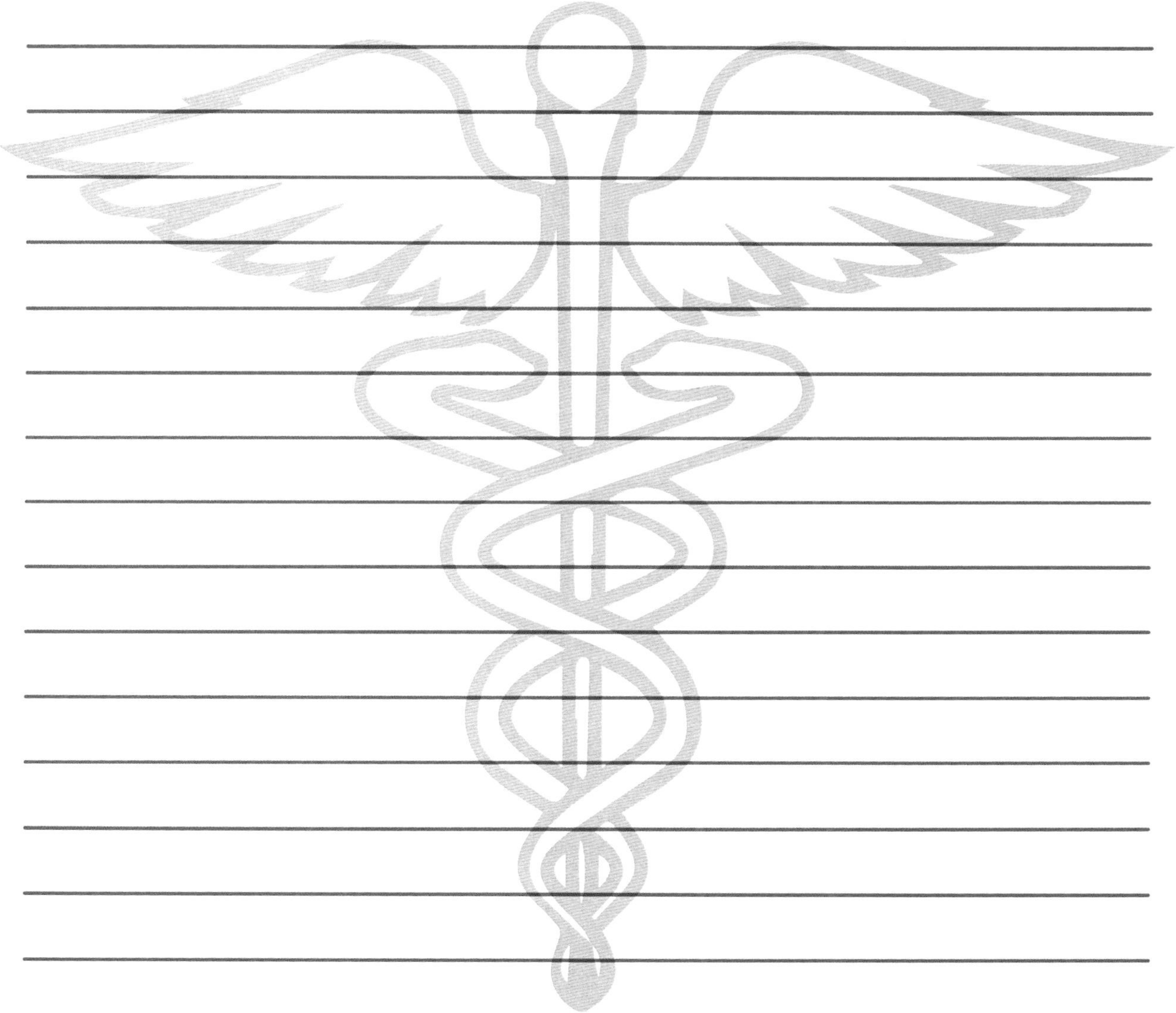

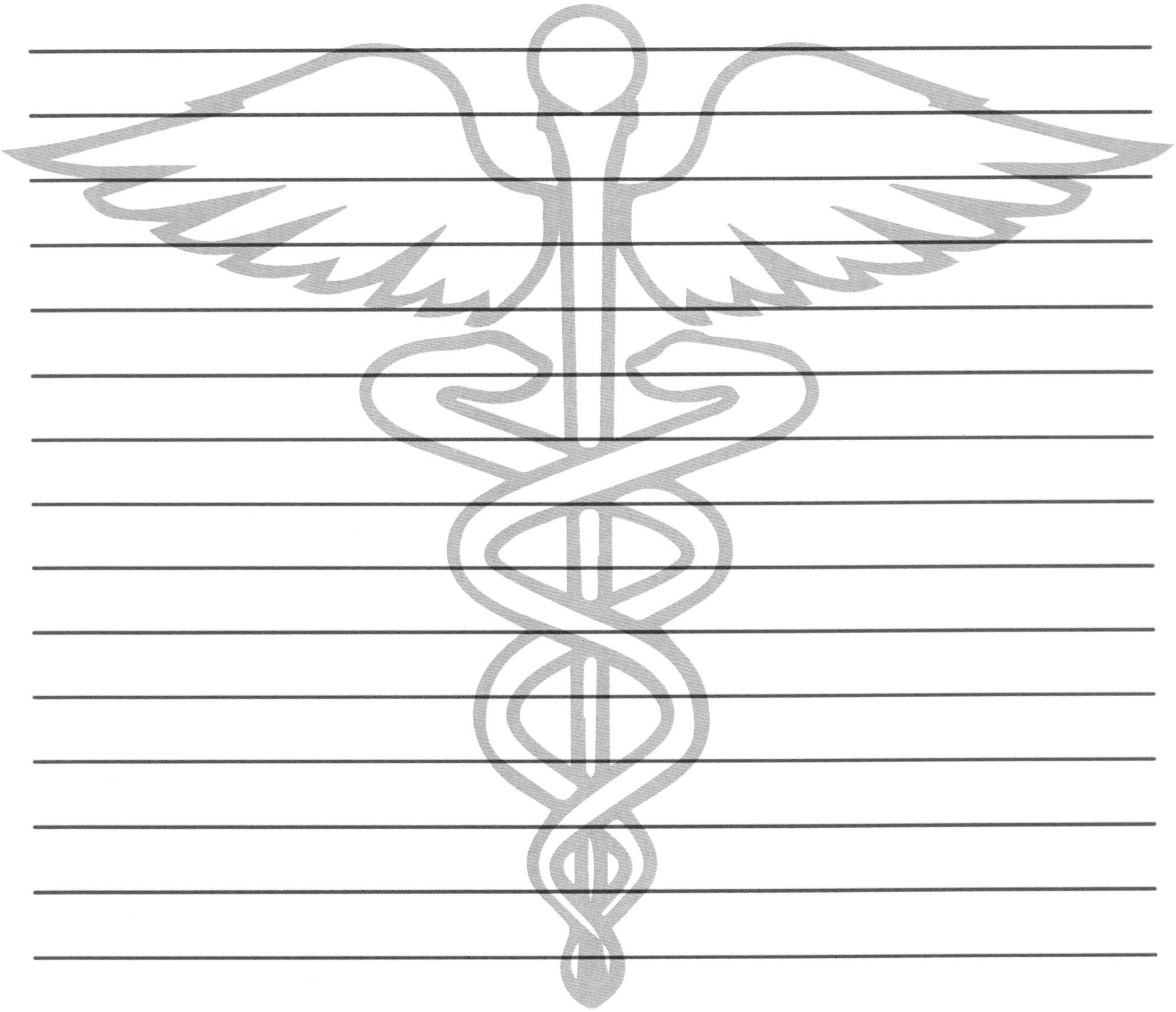

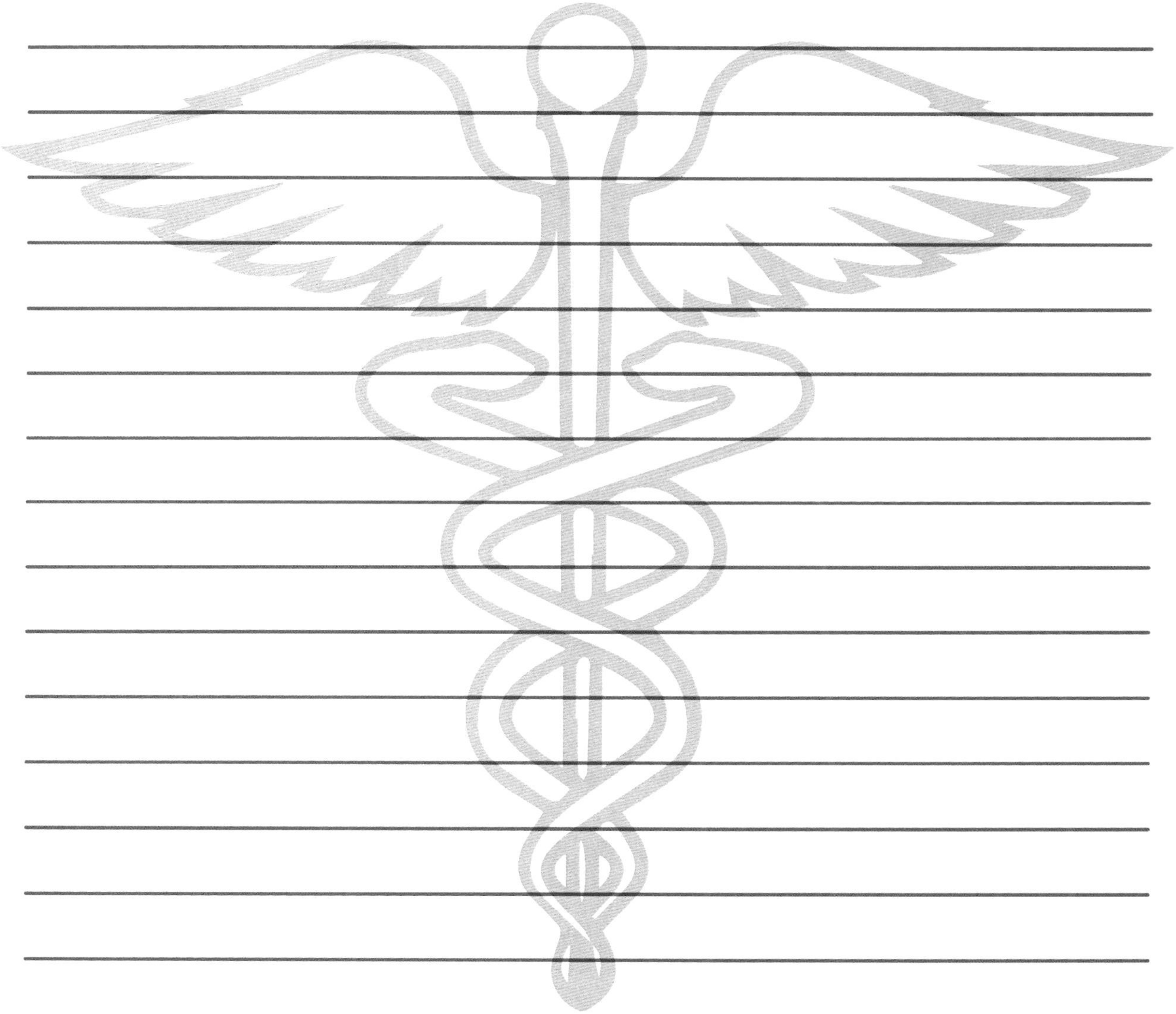

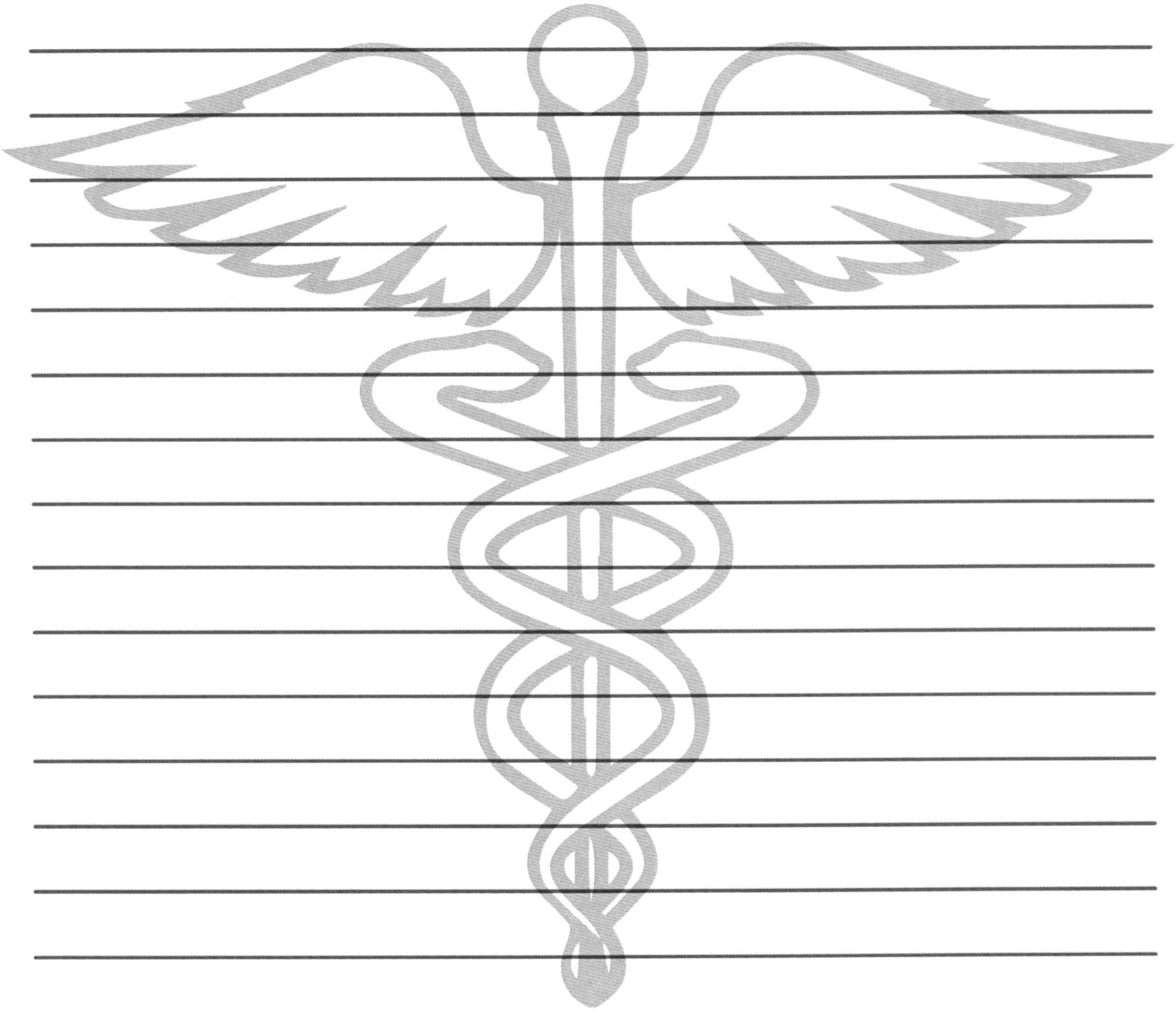

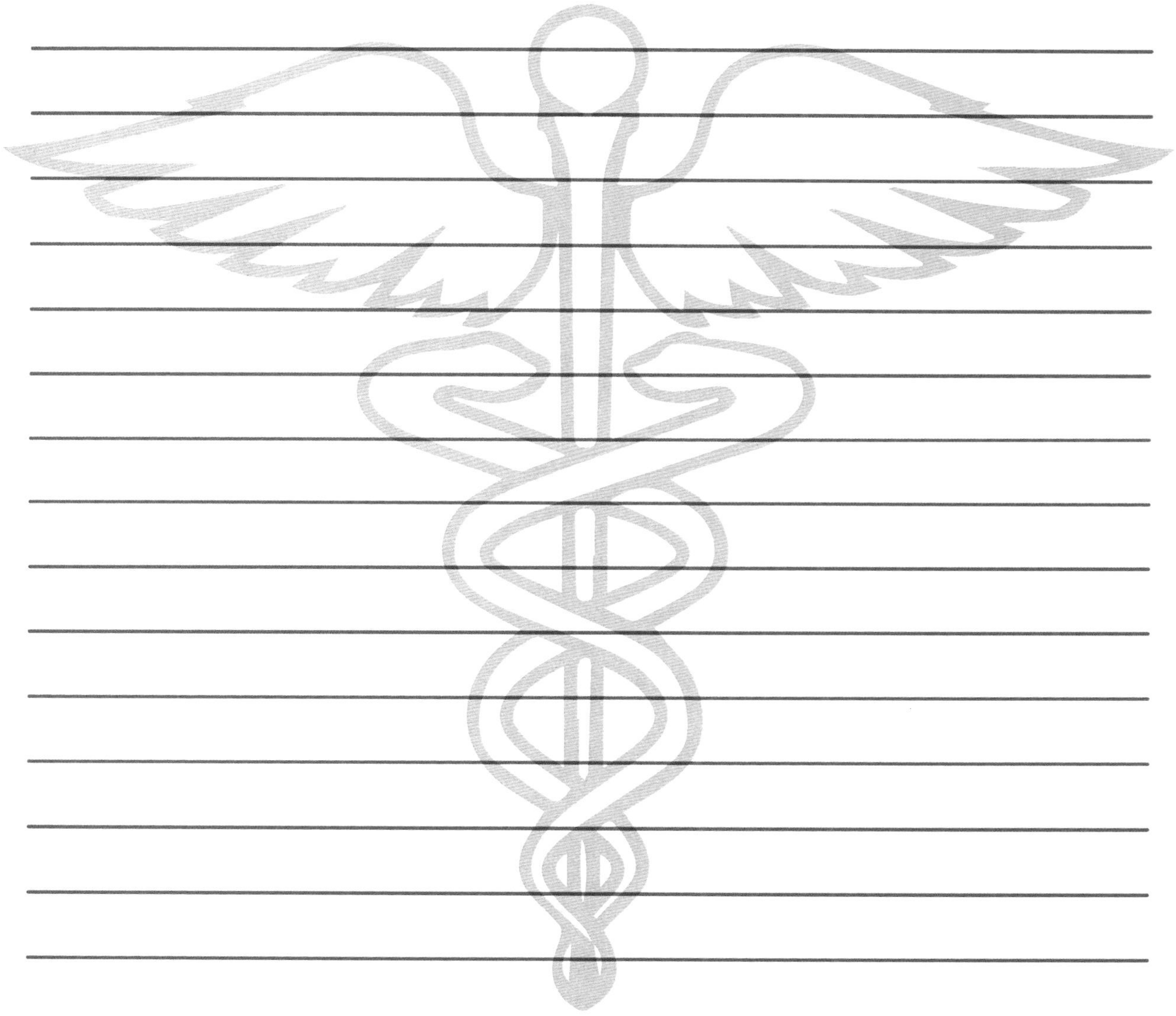

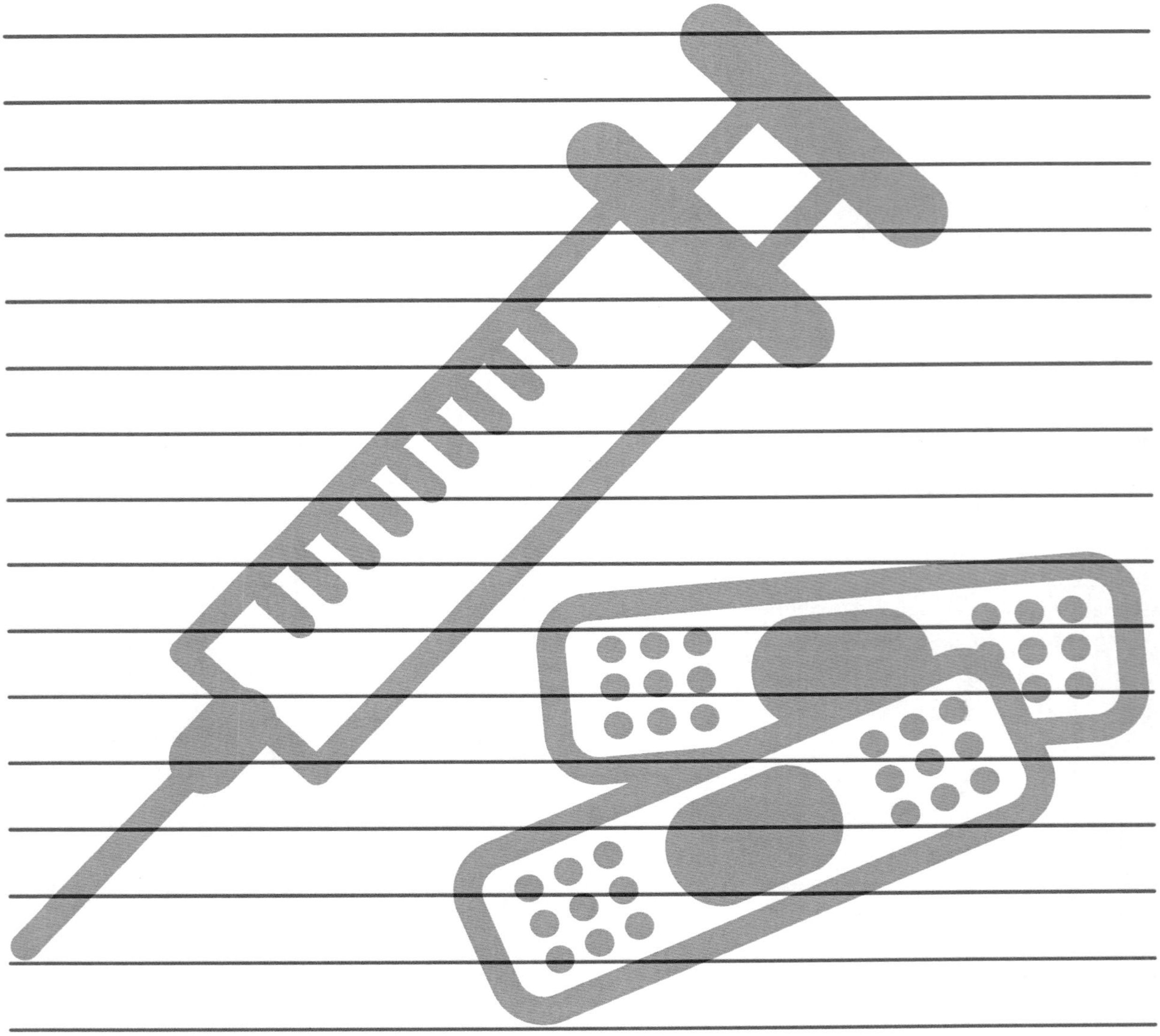

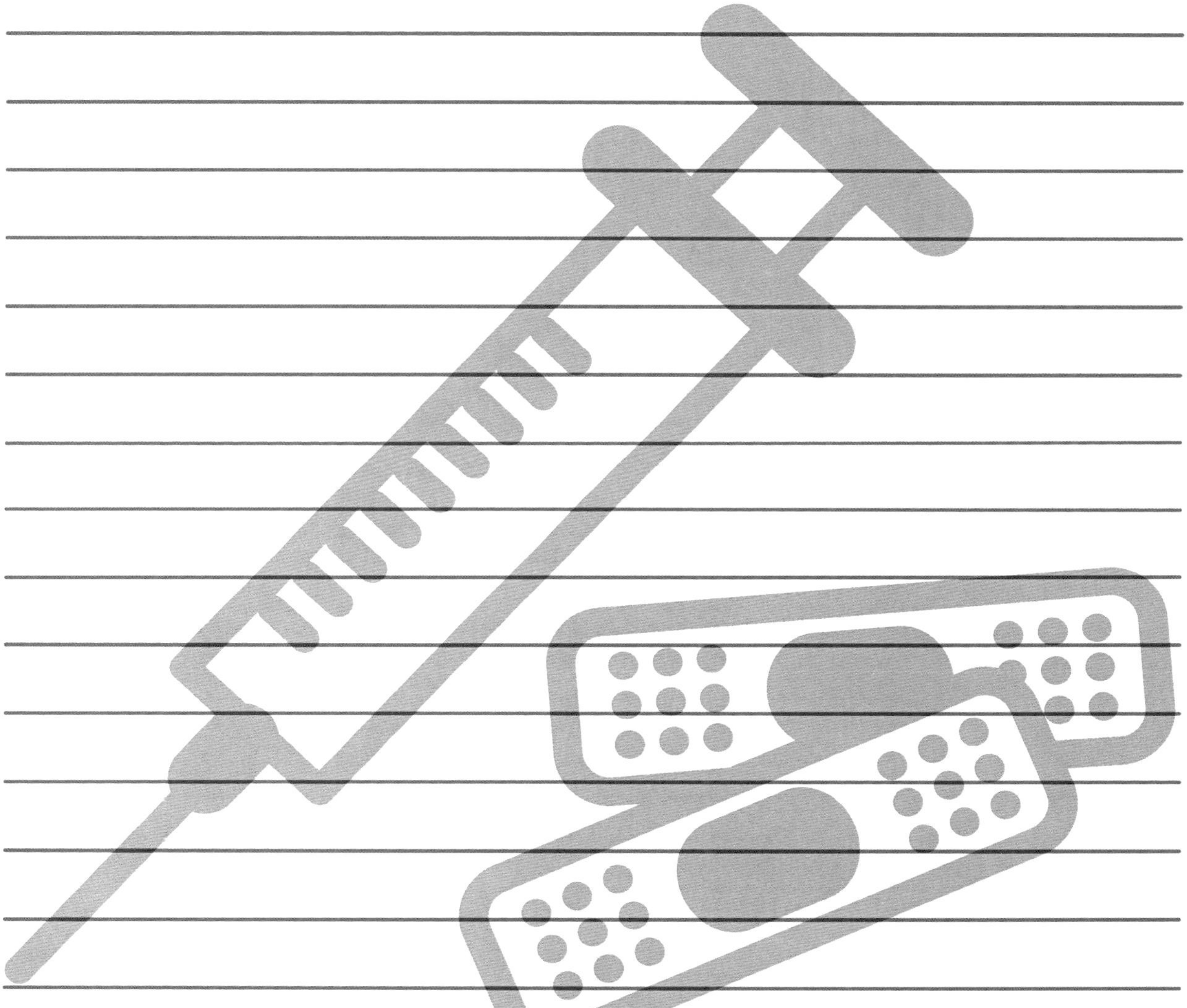

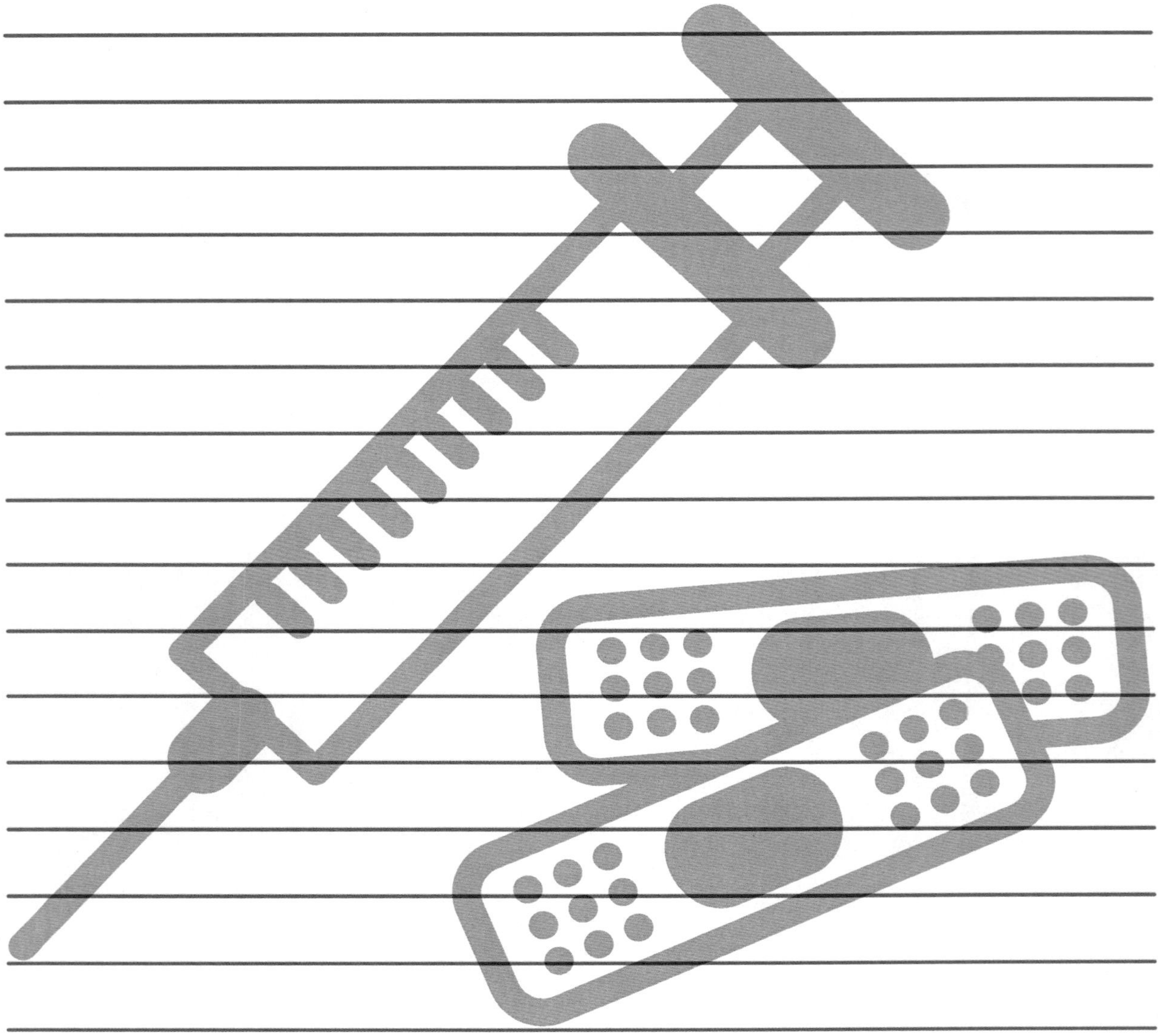

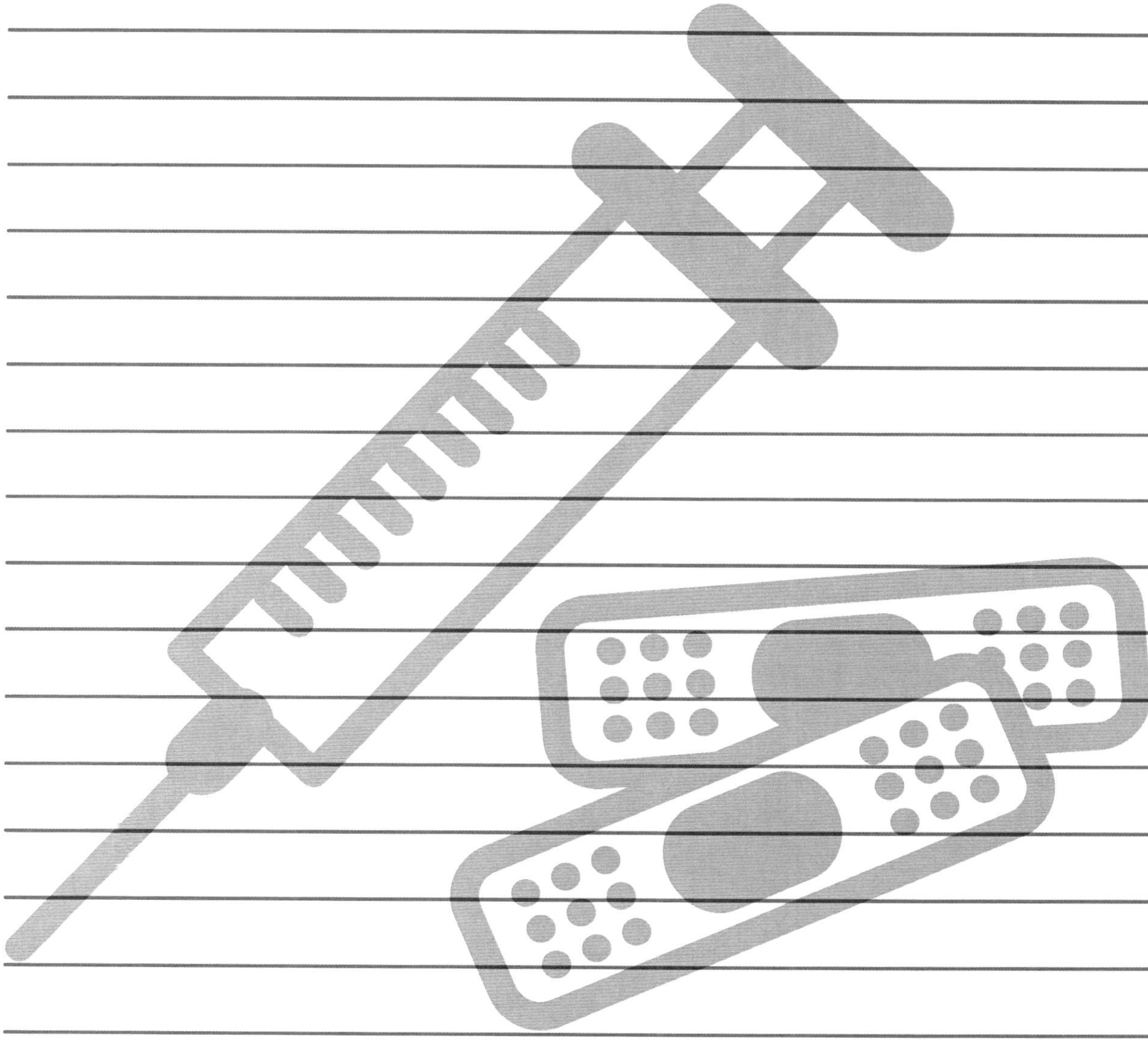

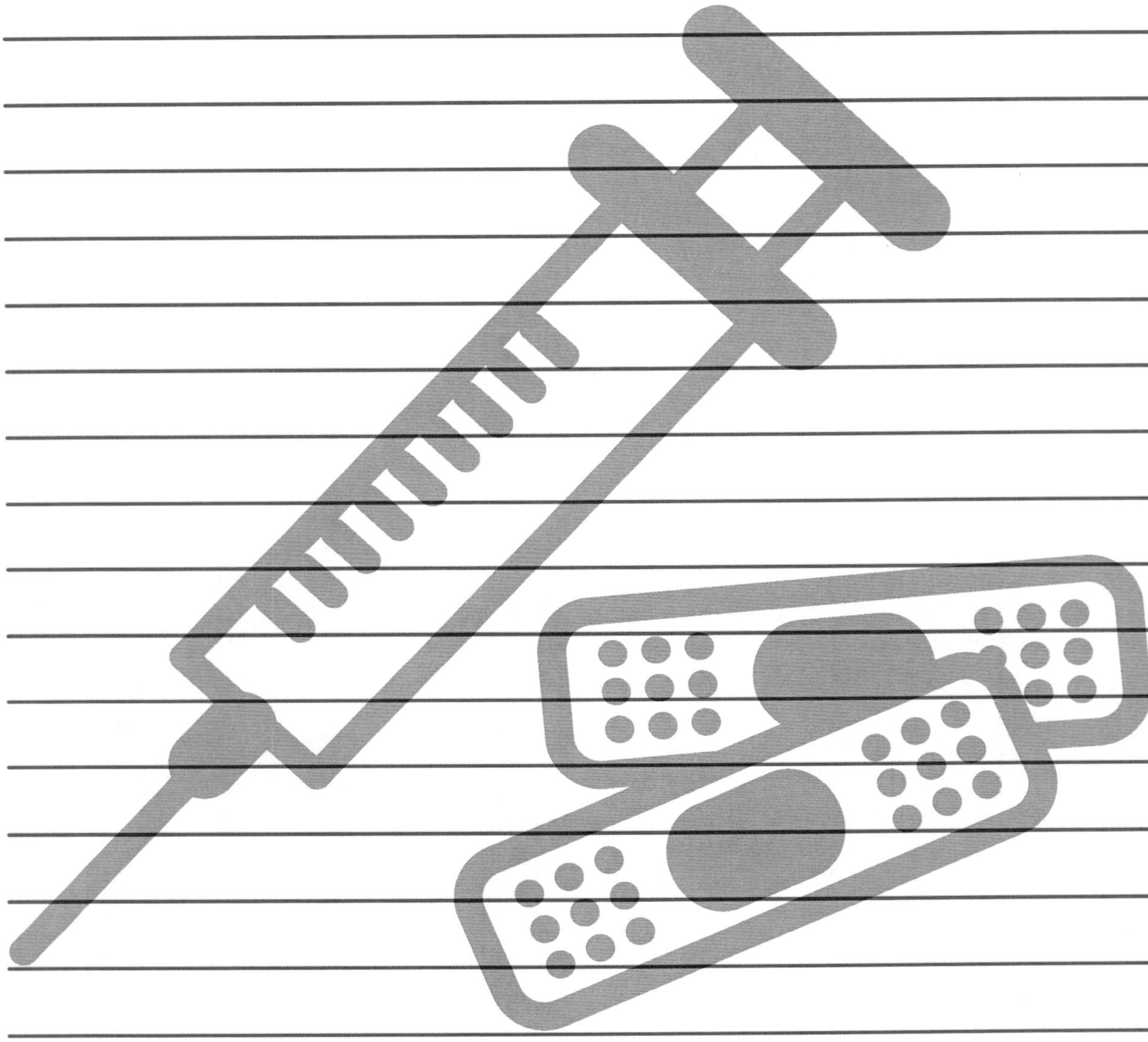

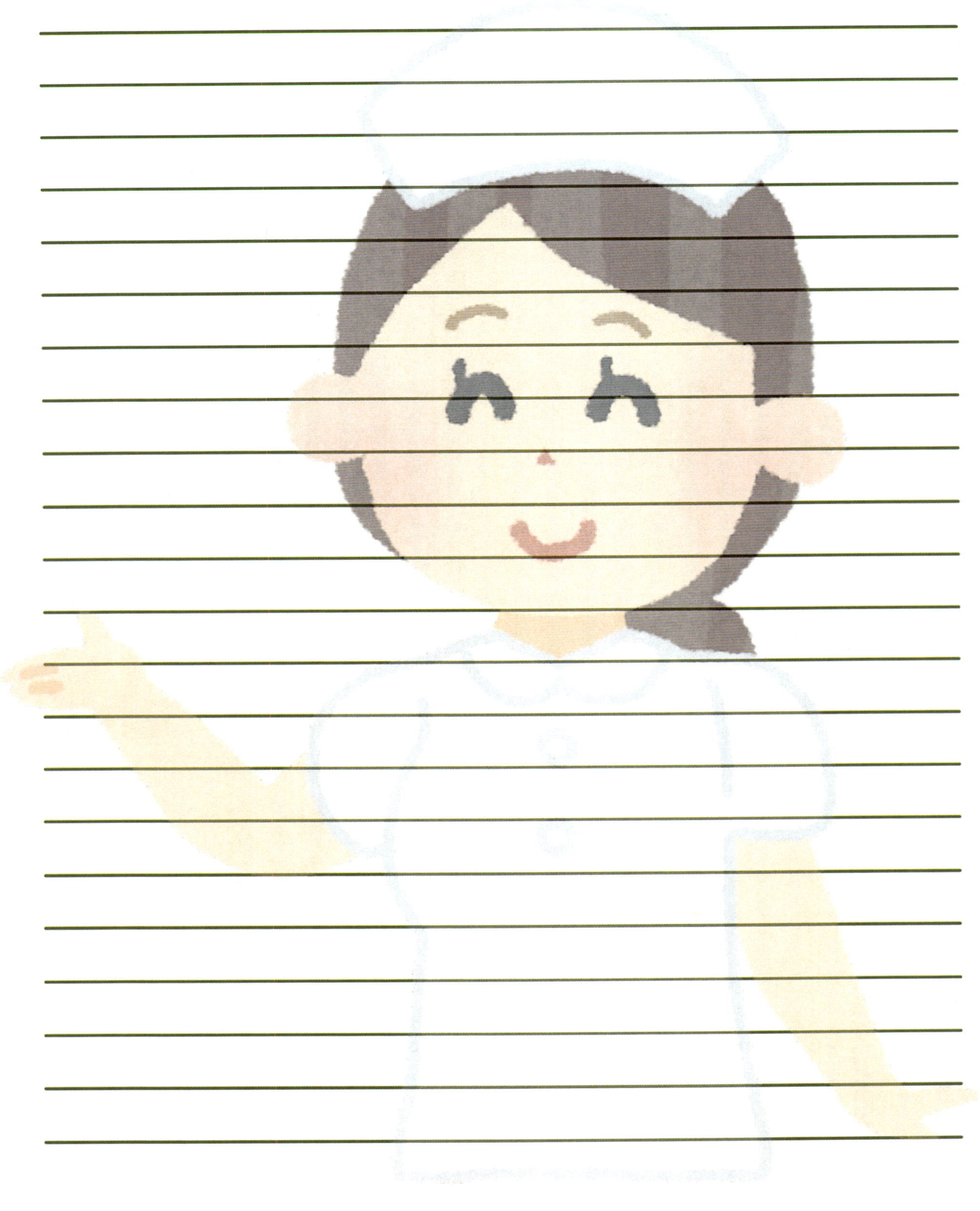

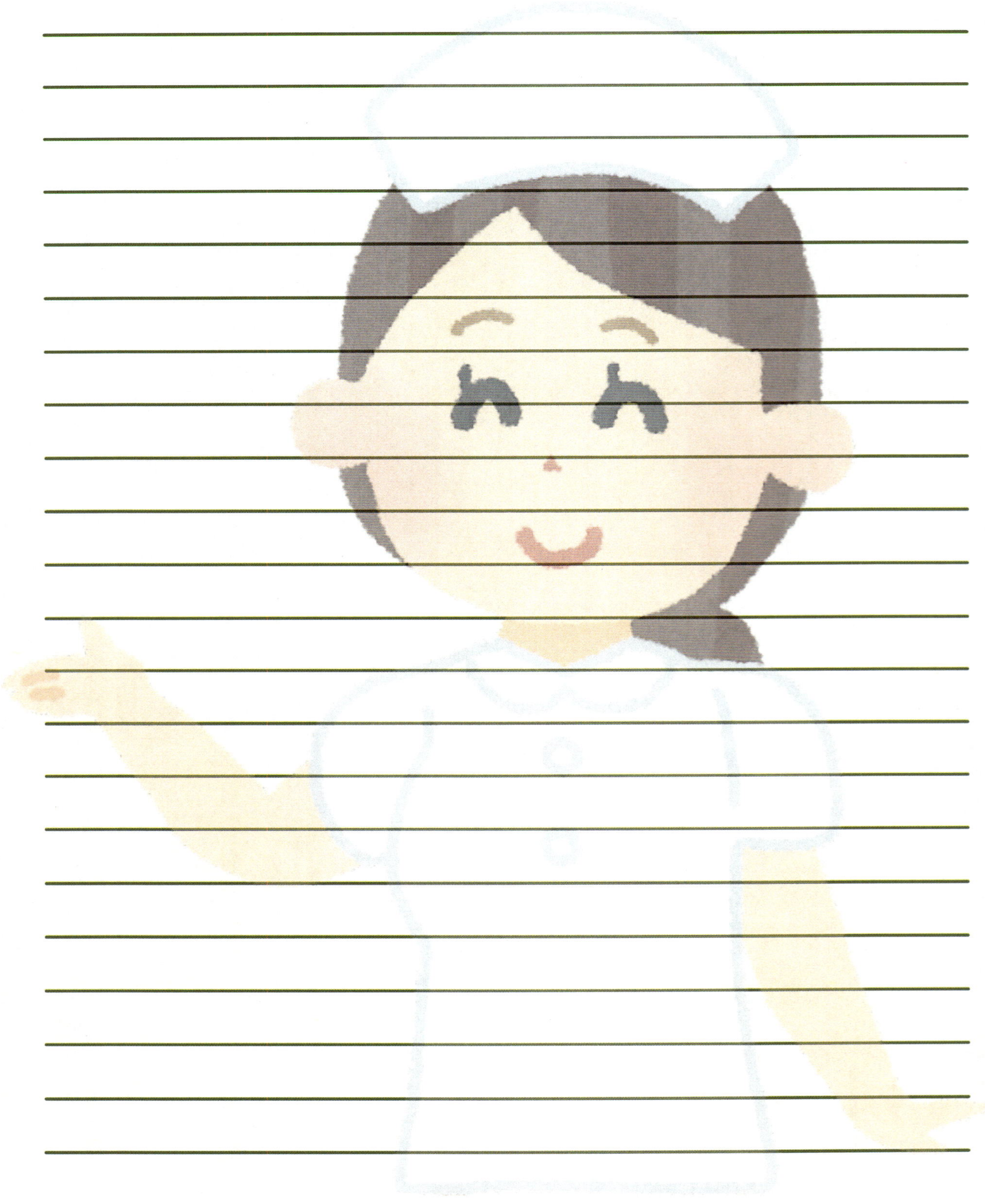

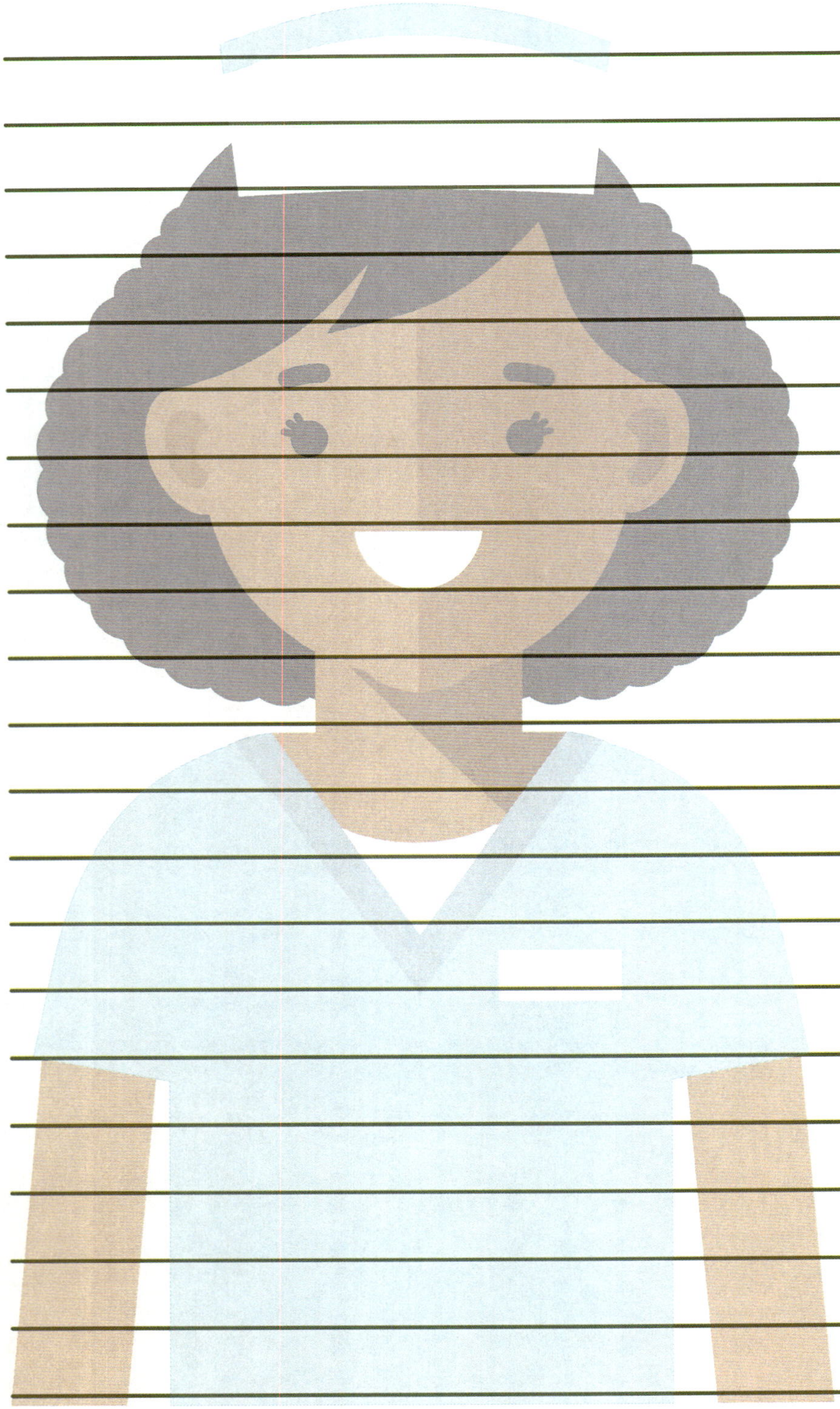

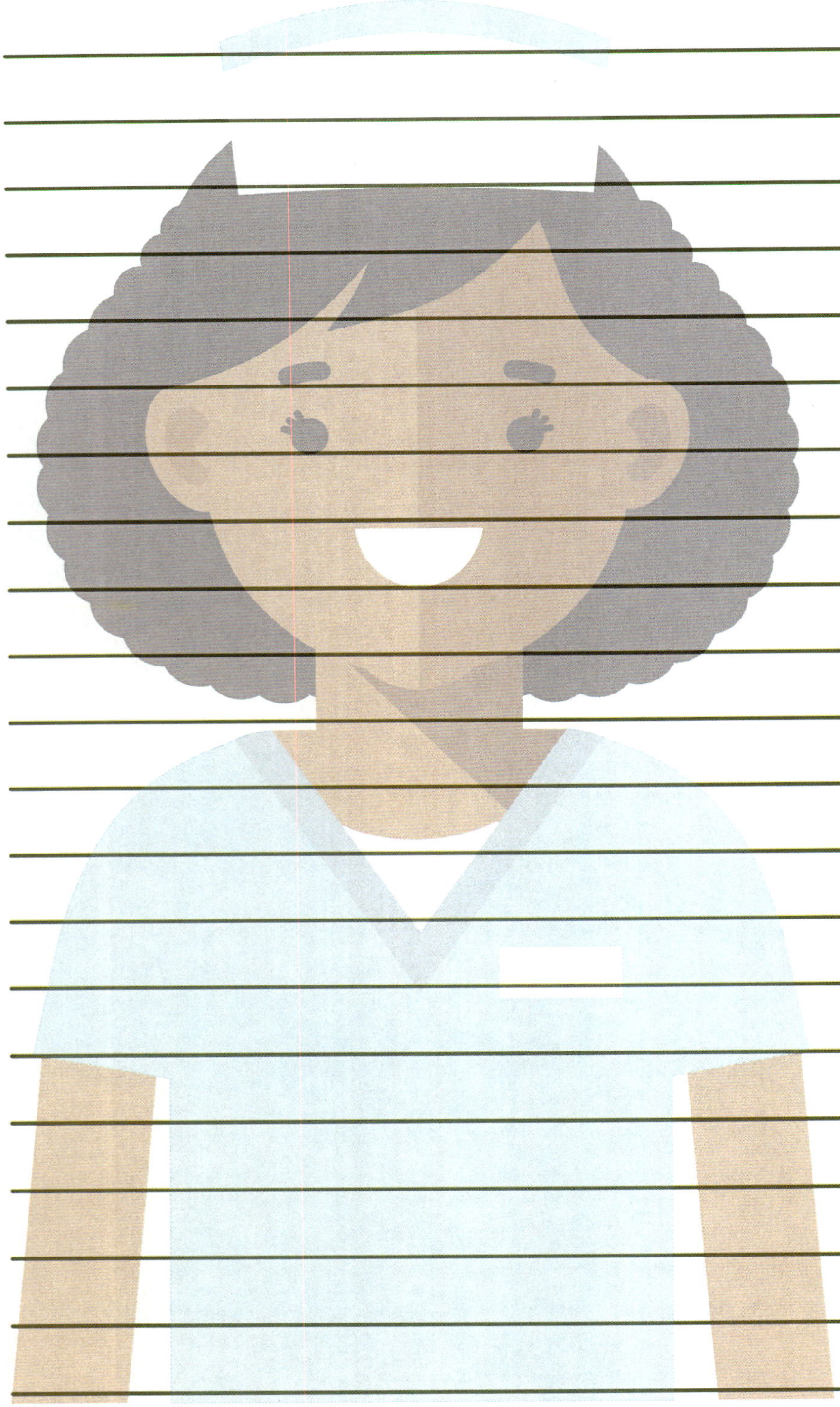

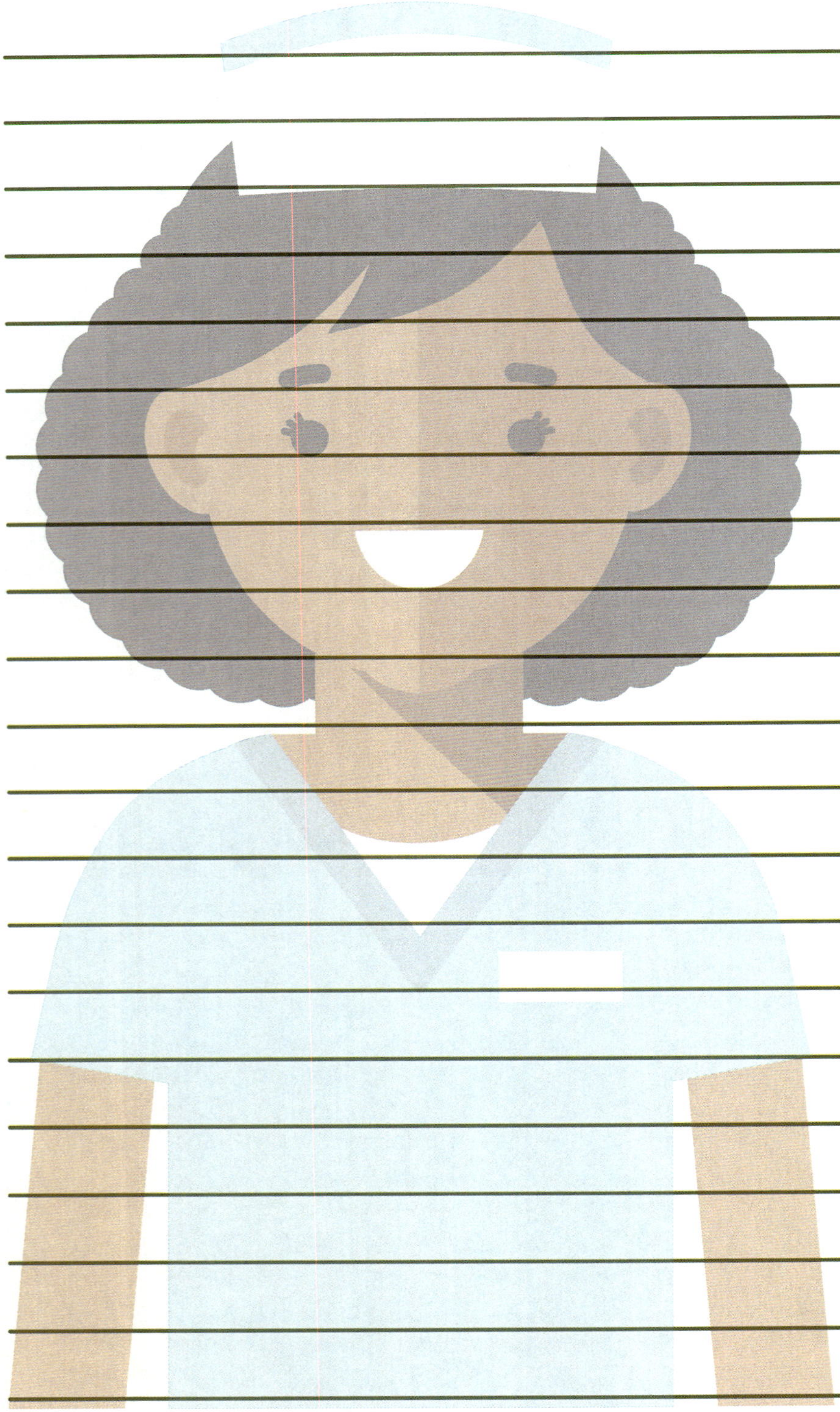

KEEP UP THE
GOOD
WORK

KEEP UP THE GOOD WORK

KEEP UP THE
GOOD
WORK

KEEP UP THE GOOD WORK

KEEP UP THE
GOOD
WORK

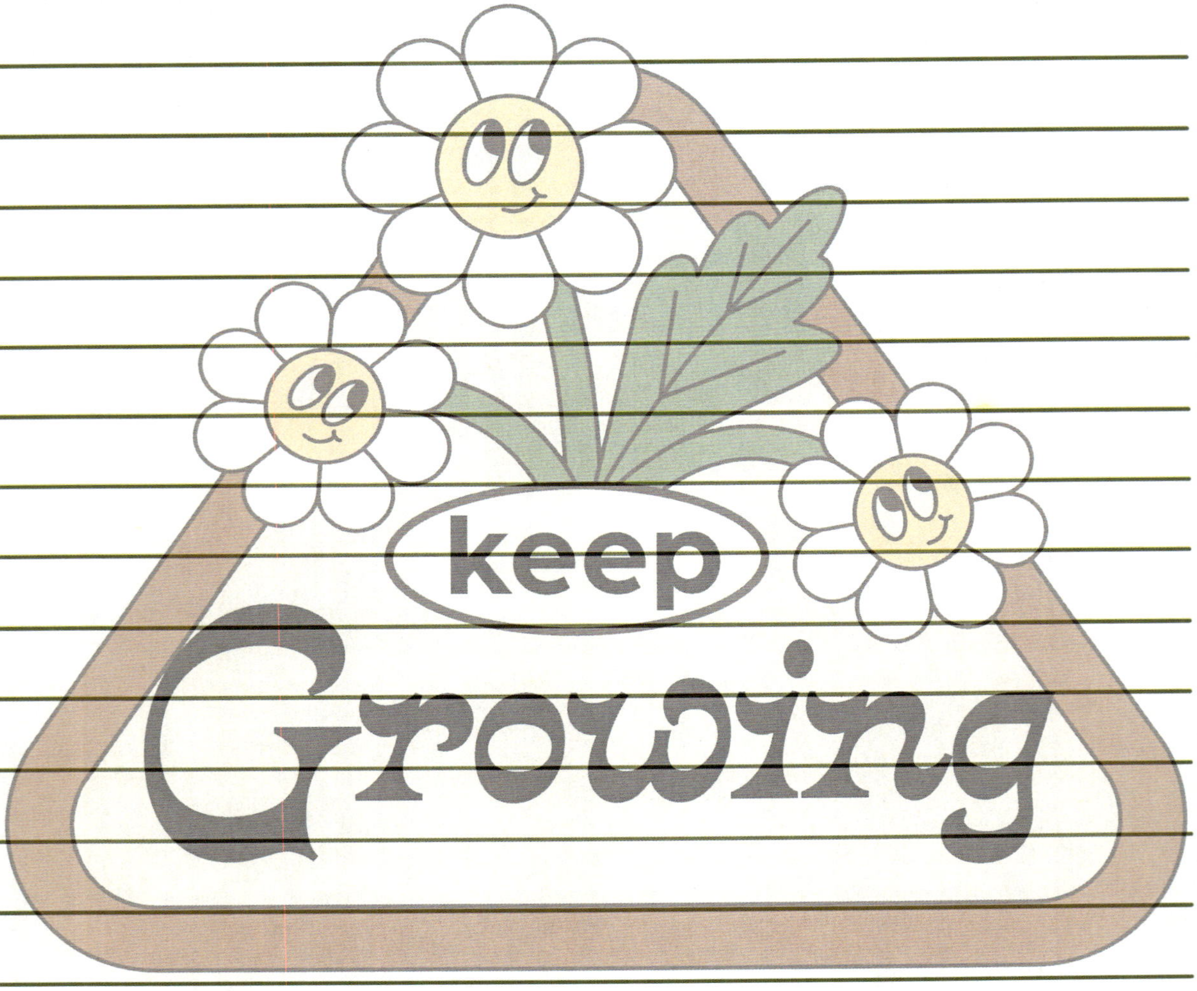
keep
Growing

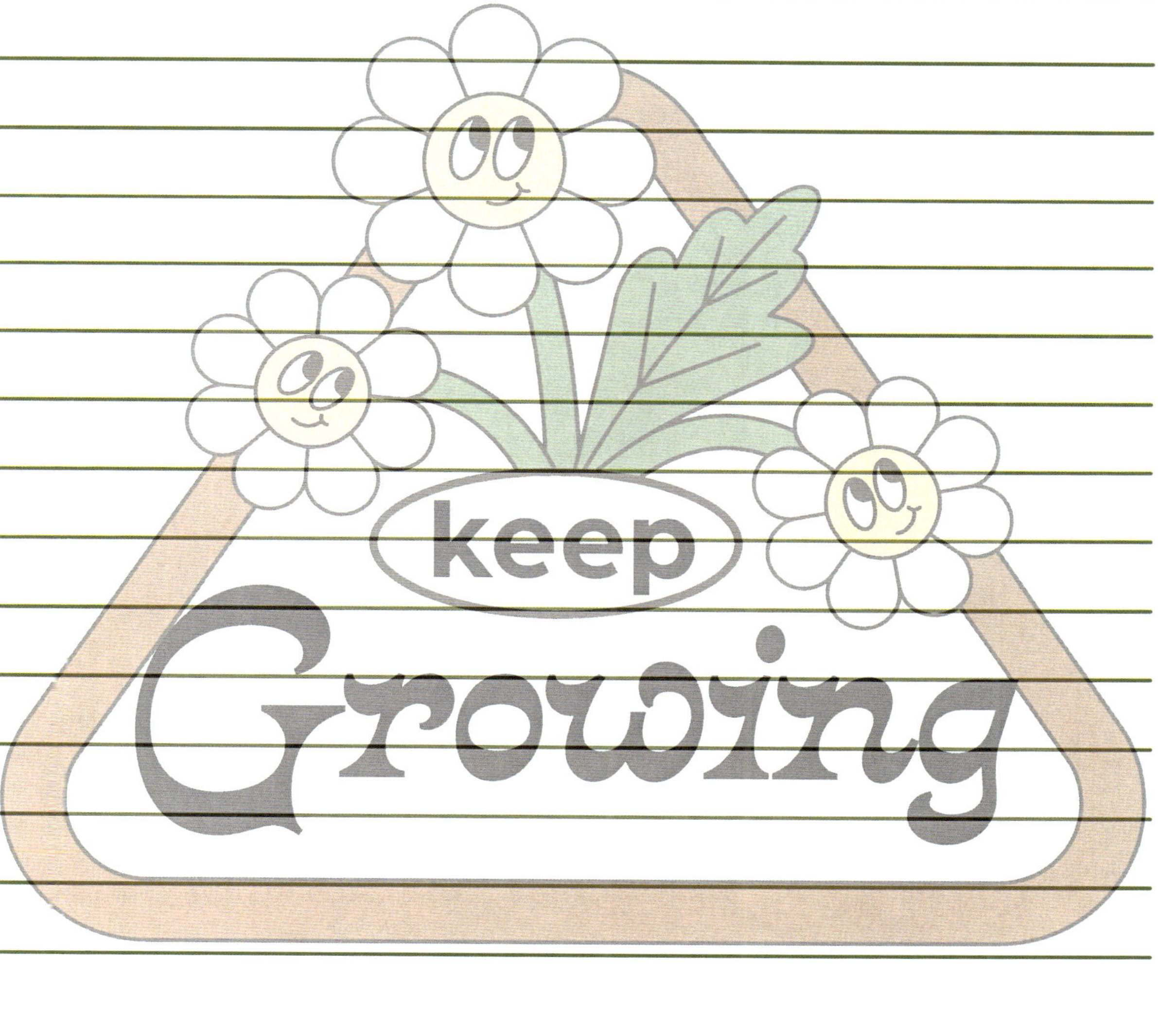
keep
Growing

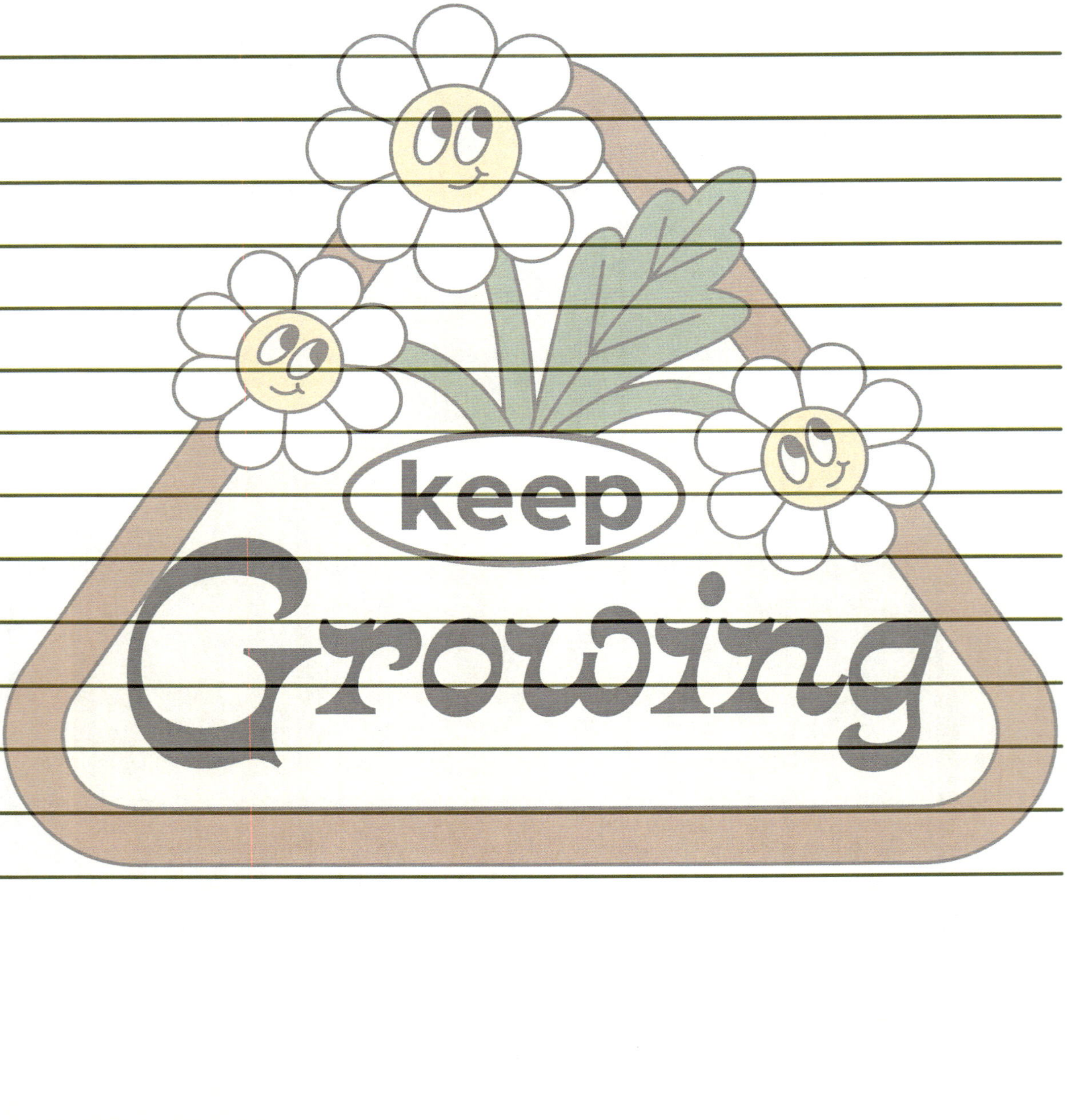
keep
Growing

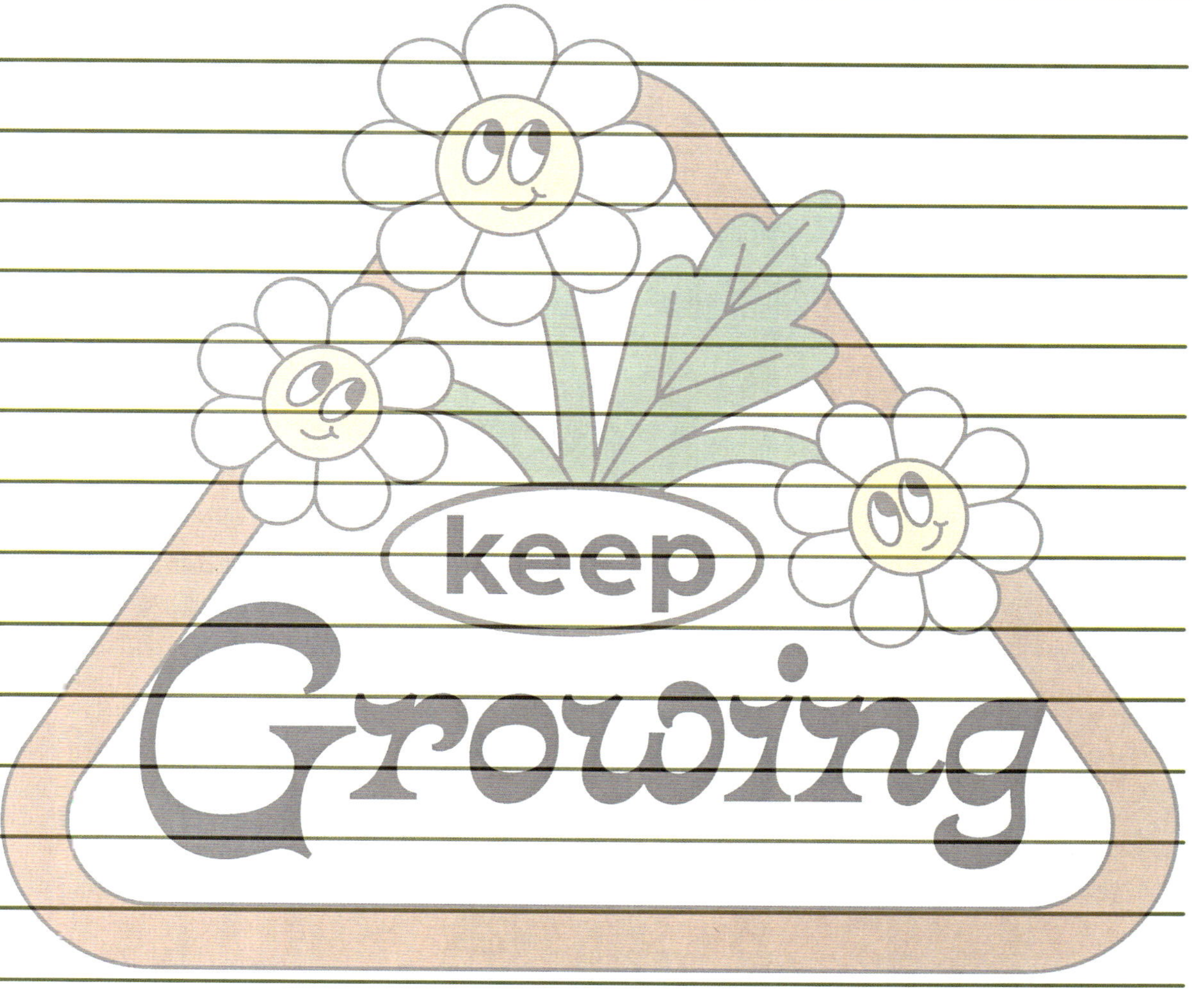
keep
Growing

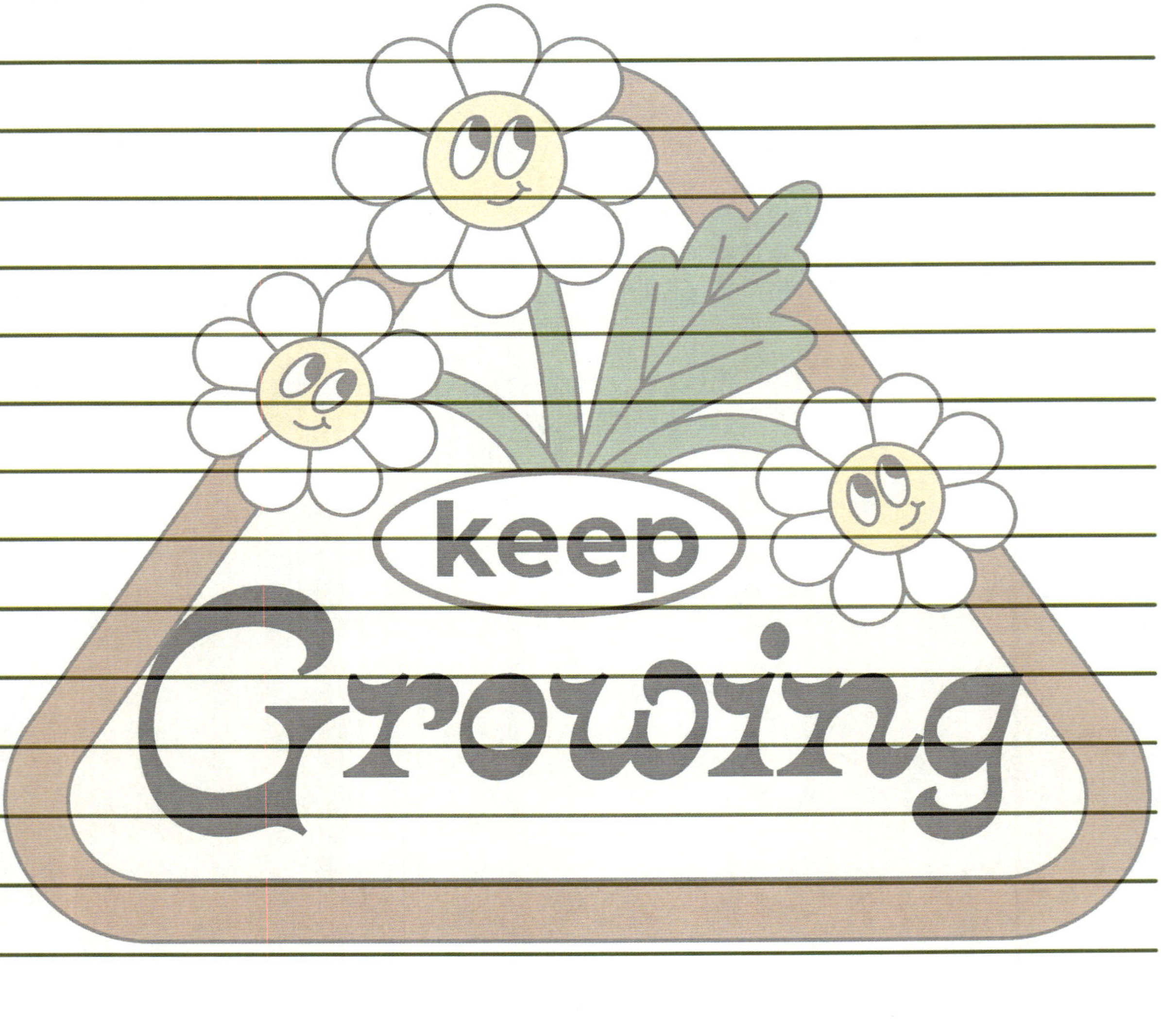
keep
Growing

KEEP FIGHTING

KEEP FIGHTING

KEEP FIGHTING

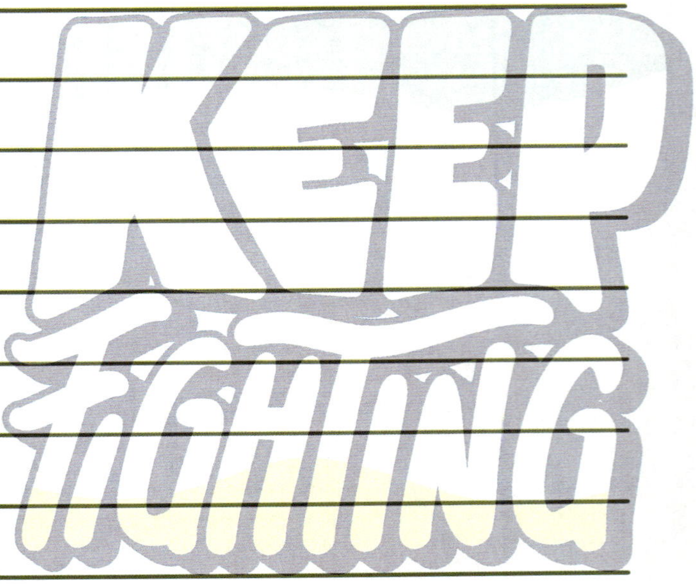
KEEP
fighting

KEEP FIGHTING

Prayer Requests

Prayer Requests

Prayer Requests

Prayer Requests

Prayer Requests

Faith

"Know therefore that the Lord your God, He is God, the faithful God, which keeps his covenant and faithfulness to a thousand generations..."

Deuteronomy 7:9 (ESV)

"If you have faith as a grain of mustard seed... nothing shall be impossible unto you."

Matthew 17:20 (ESV)

"Give thanks to the Lord, for He is good; For His faithfulness is everlasting"

1 Chronicles 16:34 (ESV)

Hope

"So do not fear, for I am with you; do not be dismayed, for I am your God. I will strengthen you and help you..."

Isaiah 41:10 (ESV)

"May the God of hope fill you with all joy and peace in believing, so that by the power of the Holy Spirit you may abound in hope."

Romans 15:13 (ESV)

"For I know the plans I have for you, declares the Lord, plans to prosper you and not to harm you; plans to give you hope and a future."

Jeremiah 29:11 (ESV)

Love

"No one has ever seen God; but if we love one another, God lives in us and His loves is made complete in us."

1 John 4:12 (ESV)

"With all humility and gentleness, with patience, bearing with one another in love, eager to maintain the unity of the Spirit..."

Ephesians 4:2-3 (ESV)

"Let the morning bring me word of your unfailing love, for I have put my trust in you. Show me the way I should go, for to you I entrust my life."

Psalm 143:8 (ESV)

Coloring Books

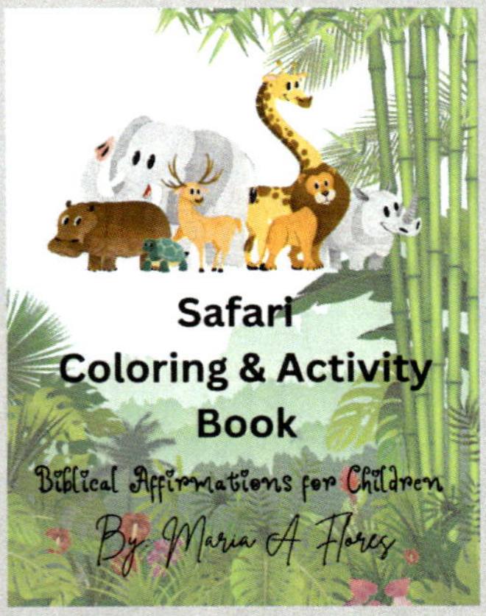

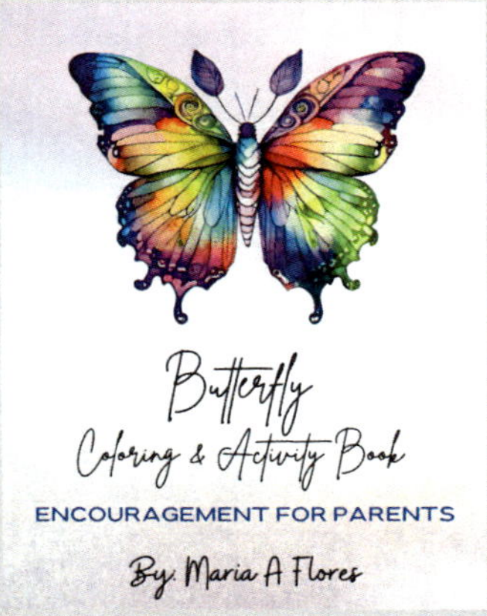

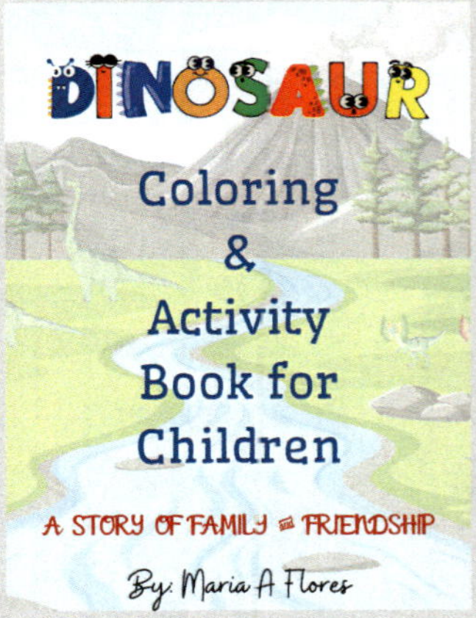

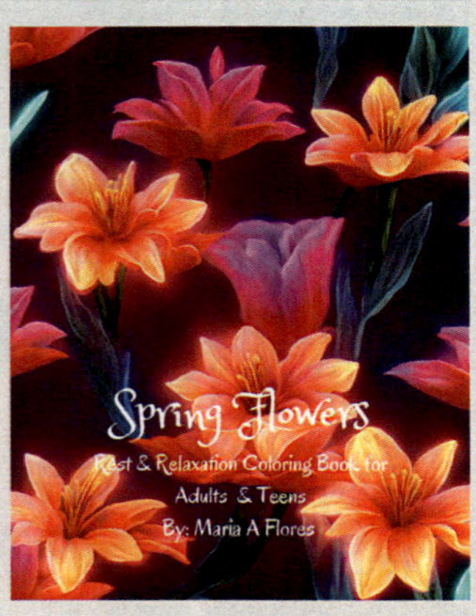

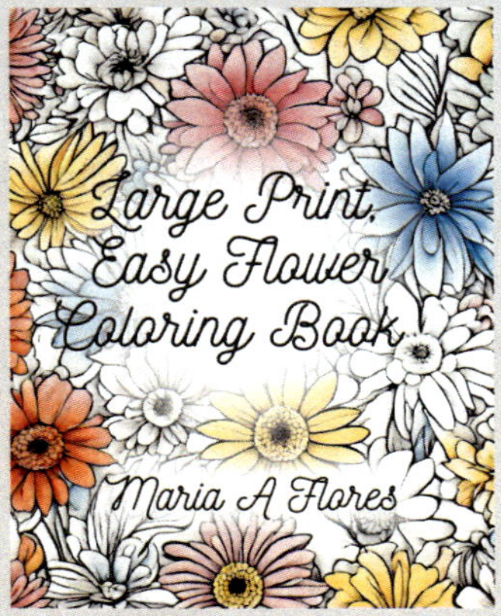

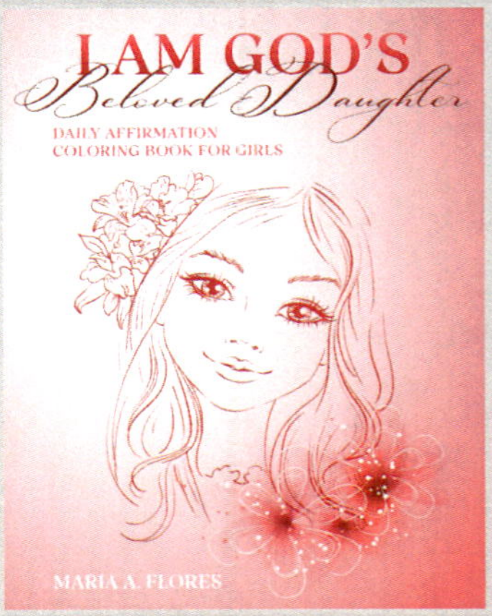

Planners

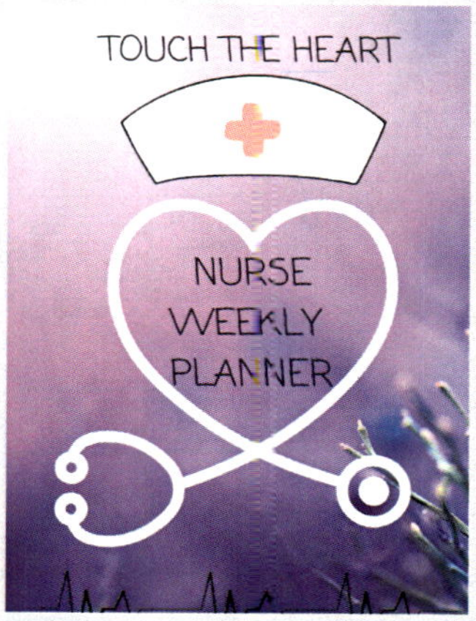
TOUCH THE HEART
NURSE
WEEKLY
PLANNER

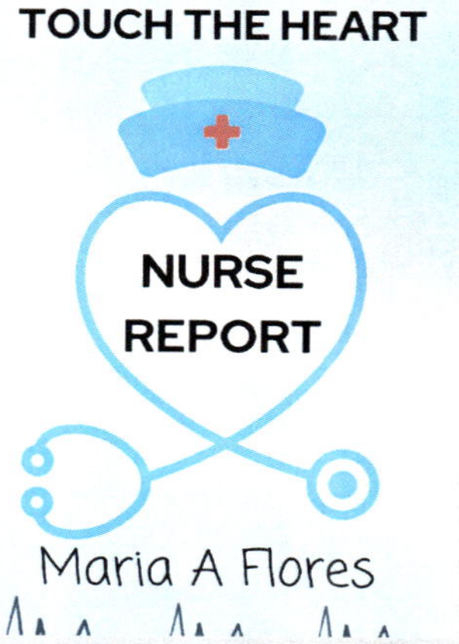
TOUCH THE HEART
NURSE
REPORT
Maria A Flores

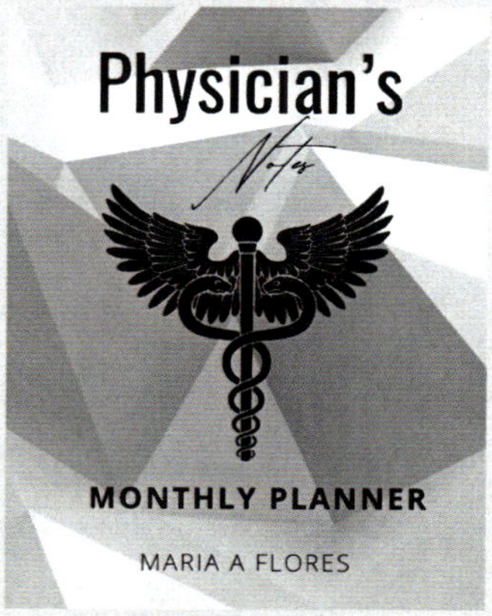
Physician's
MONTHLY PLANNER
MARIA A FLORES

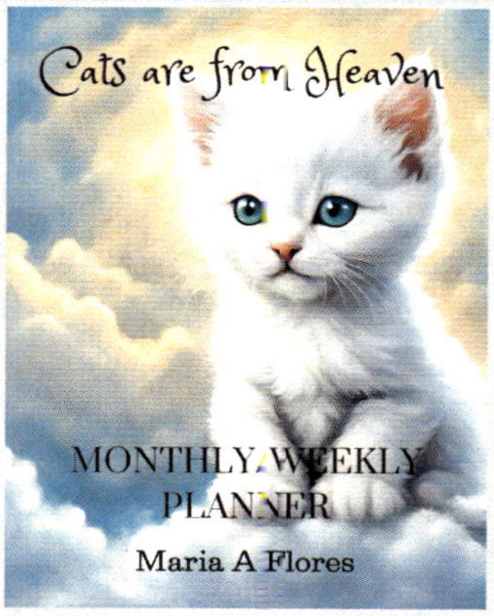
Cats are from Heaven
MONTHLY WEEKLY
PLANNER
Maria A Flores

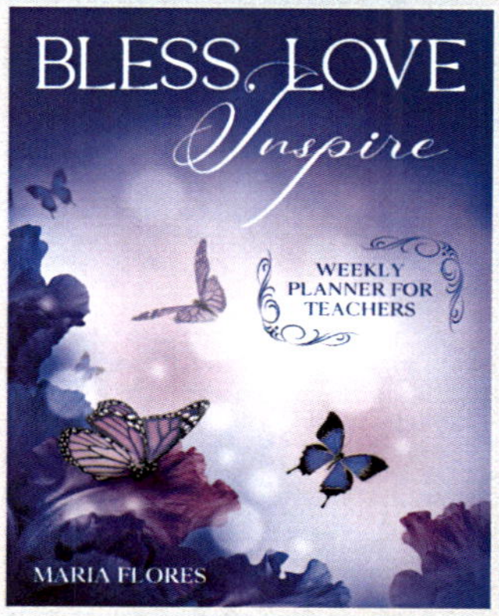
BLESS LOVE
Inspire
WEEKLY
PLANNER FOR
TEACHERS
MARIA FLORES

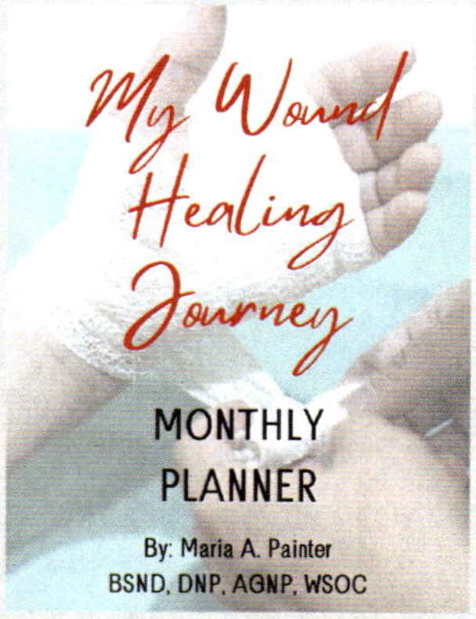
My Wound
Healing
Journey
MONTHLY
PLANNER
By: Maria A. Painter
BSND, DNP, AGNP, WSOC

Notebooks

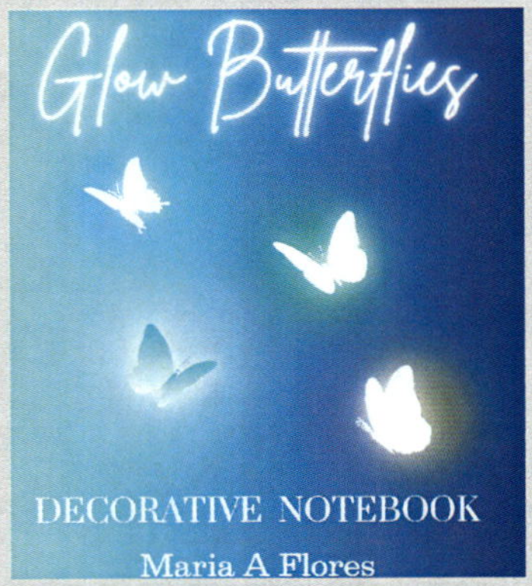
Glow Butterflies
DECORATIVE NOTEBOOK
Maria A Flores

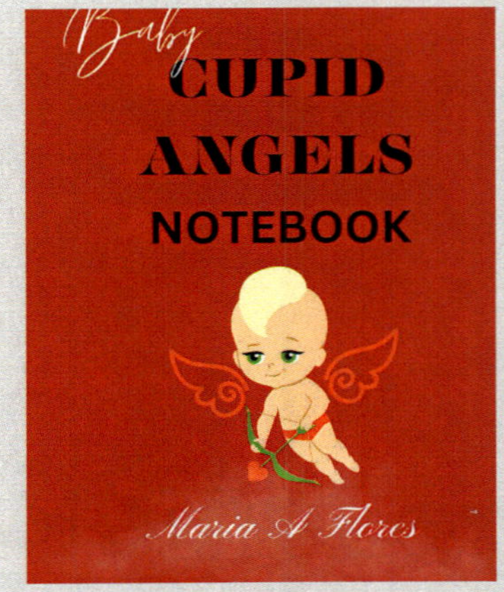
Baby
CUPID
ANGELS
NOTEBOOK
Maria A Flores

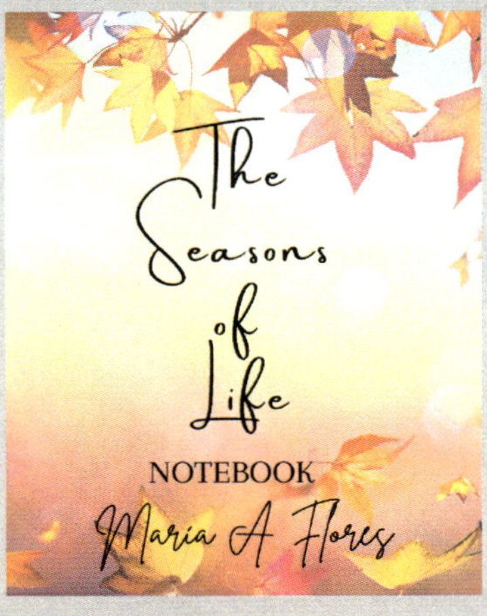
The
Seasons
of
Life
NOTEBOOK
Maria A Flores

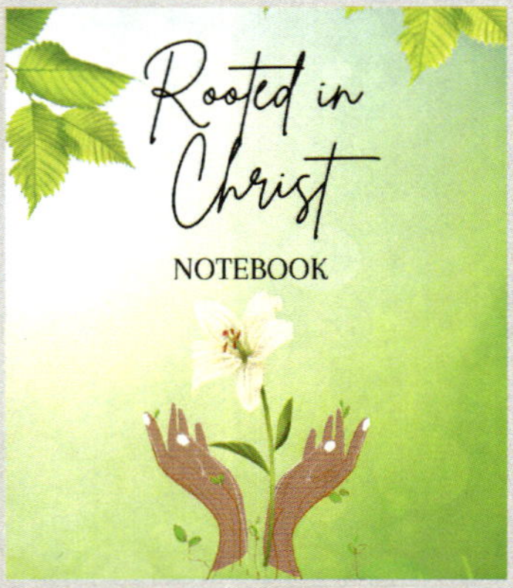
Rooted in
Christ
NOTEBOOK

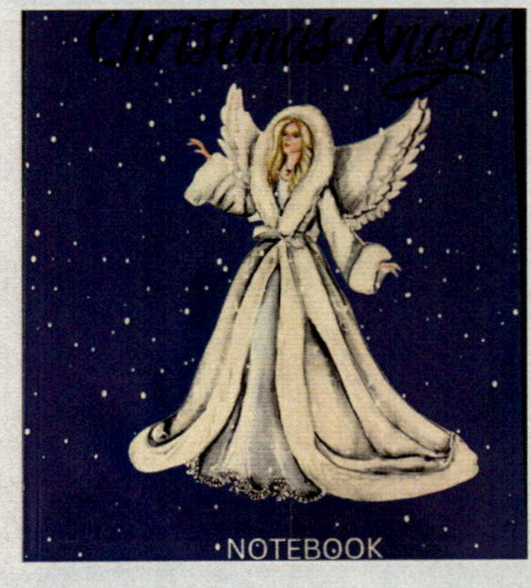
Christmas Angels
NOTEBOOK

Journals

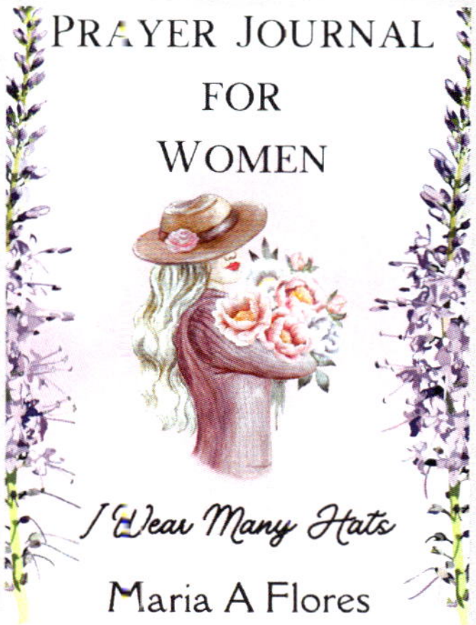

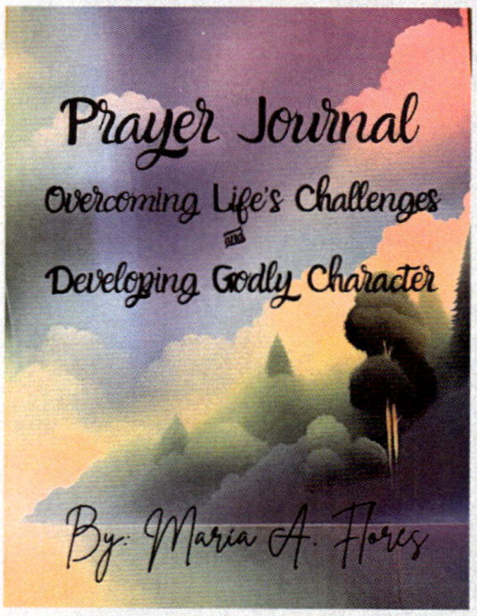

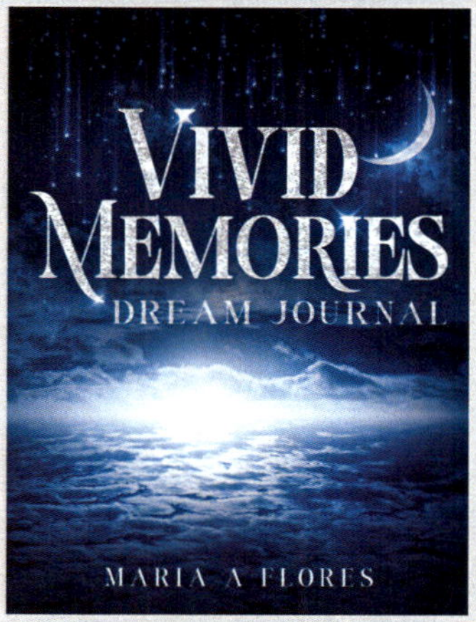

For God so loved the world that he gave his only begotten son, that whosoever believes in Him should not perish, but have everlasting life (John 3:16).

http://touchtheheartreachthesoul.store

Made in United States
North Haven, CT
06 November 2026

21765024R20069